Chocolate
Unwrapped

CHOCOLATE UNWRAPPED

The Surprising Health Benefits *of* America's Favorite Passion

ROWAN JACOBSEN

INVISIBLE CITIES PRESS
MONTPELIER, VERMONT

Invisible Cities Press
50 State Street
Montpelier, VT 05602
www.invisiblecitiespress.com

Library of Congress Cataloging-in-Publication Data
Jacobsen, Rowan.
  Chocolate unwrapped : the surprising health benefits of America's
favorite passion / Rowan Jacobsen.
    p.   cm.
Includes bibliographical references and index.
  ISBN 1-931229-31-7
  1. Chocolate—Health aspects. I. Title.
  QP144.C46J33 2003
  613.2'84—dc21

                              2003013537

Printed in Canada on 100 percent post-consumer recycled paper

Book design by Peter Holm, Sterling Hill Productions

Photographs courtesy of the Chocolate Manufacturers Association.

Contents

INTRODUCTION 1

1. **A Brief History of Chocolate** 8

2. **From Bean to Bonbon** 22

    Dark Chocolate 29

    Milk Chocolate 31

    Cocoa Powder 32

    The Proof Is in the Pudding 33

3. **Chocolate *Is* Health Food** 34

    What Are Antioxidants? 35

    Top Antioxidant Foods 36

    How Antioxidants Work 37

    The Panama Paradox 40

    Tasty Aspirin? 41

    Chocolate Studies 42

    Other Antioxidant Studies 43

        Cardiovascular Disease 43

        Cancer 45

        Alzheimer's Disease 46

        Arthritis 47

        Asthma and Allergies 48

        Cough Suppressant 48

    The Big Picture 49

4. **What's in Chocolate?** 50

    The Skinny on Fat 50

    Chocolate Nutrients 54

        Nutrient Information of Dark Chocolate 55

    Cocoa Content 58

5. **Chocolate on the Brain** 61

    Caffeine 62

    Theobromine 63

    Serotonin and Tryptophan 64

    Phenylethylamine 65

    Anandamide 66

    The Perfect Storm 68

    Cravings 69

6. **Melting the Myths** 72

    Acne 73

    Allergies 74

    ADHD 75

    Cavities 76

    Heart Palpitations 77

    Migraines 77

    Obesity 79

7. **Chocolate Growing Today:** *Child Labor and Environmental Issues* 80

    Labor Practices 81

    Environmental Issues 85

8. **Recipes** 89

    Chocolate Sauce 91

    Chocolate Tandoori 92

    Chocolate Corn Bread 94

Mary's Holy Mole 96

Sicilian Chocolate Pasta 98

New World Nachos 100

Chocolate Breakfast Atole 101

Grown-up Hot Chocolate 102

Righteous Cookies 104

Not-Messing-Around Chocolate Cake 106

World's Best Brownies 108

Simple Chocolate Mousse 110

Enrobed Bananas 112

CONCLUSION: *Chocolate Is Not Sinful* 113

RESOURCES: *The World's Healthiest, Most Delicious*
Chocolate, Delivered to Your Door 115

Chocolate Companies 115

Mail Order 121

Magazines 122

Informational Websites 122

ACKNOWLEDGMENTS 124

REFERENCES 125

Introduction

If you are like me, you grew up loving chocolate, but feeling a bit guilty whenever you ate it. Chocolate was indescribably delicious—nobody argued with that—but it was just somehow *bad* for you. Was it the fat? The sugar? The reasons were never entirely clear. What was clear, however, was that chocolate was a treat, something to be consumed only after you had eaten enough "good" food to offset the evil effects of the chocolate, whatever they were. I thought of chocolate as a guilty pleasure, a sinful indulgence.

What I had no way of knowing—what few people knew back then—was that chocolate had been revered as a sacred, indispensable, and healthy food by the Maya and Aztecs for thousands of years. I just knew that I felt good after eating it. Satisfied, alert, and happy.

Today, we know that the chocolate was bathing my brain in natural endorphins, just as it was for those Maya. Not only that, but it was keeping my heart, blood vessels, brain, and teeth healthy. This was undoubtedly part of the reason why the Maya held chocolate in such esteem. They lovingly tended groves of cacao in the rainforest, called it "the food of the gods," and used it in both their daily life and their most holy ceremonies. They would have been horrified to see the way Europeans took this natural health food and cut it with so much cream and sugar that it became famously naughty to eat.

The story of how chocolate's reputation transformed from sacred food to guilty pleasure, and why it is beginning to change back again, is the subject of this book. Thanks to the increasingly sophisticated American palate, and to the latest in dietary science, we are again learning what the ancients knew for millennia: not only is chocolate divine, but it's also very good for you.

You're skeptical. Chocolate? *Good* for us? Seems unlikely. Yet a host of recent studies shows that chocolate reduces our risk of heart disease and stroke, and may prevent cancers and other diseases, too. Scientists are still trying to determine exactly how chocolate does this, but it stems from the fact that chocolate is absolutely loaded with antioxidants, the same compounds that make fruit, red wine, and green tea good for you.

Because chocolate is made from the seeds of a fruit, it should be no surprise that it is full of antioxidants, as are most fruits. The seeds come in ten-inch-long, football-shaped pods that grow directly from the trunk of the cacao tree *(Theobroma cacao),* which thrives only in tropical regions and probably originated in Mesoamerica. (*Cacao* refers to the plant, including the pods and seeds, in its natural form, while *cocoa* indicates the pure product derived from cacao beans, and *chocolate* refers to the final form, whether drink or solid.) Cacao is as natural and

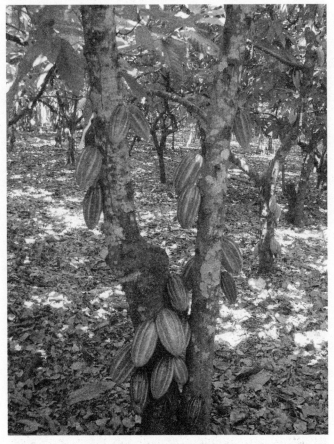

Theobroma cacao, in all its glory.

healthy as any fruit, and was consumed as an unsweetened drink for its culinary, stimulating, and healing properties by the Olmec, Maya, and Aztecs for thousands of years before it was ever discovered by Europeans, who also consumed chocolate almost exclusively in drink form until late in the nineteenth century.

But here's the rub. Notice that those early civilizations consumed chocolate as an *unsweetened* drink. The Maya's only sources of sweetener were honey or sap from the maguey cactus, and neither was in great supply. They drank their chocolate bitter and liked it that way. The Spanish saw things differently. They shared the dark, spicy drink with their New World hosts and thought, "Yeck! Needs cream and sugar." Since then, we've come to associate the taste of chocolate with the flavor of the sugar and milk invariably added to it, and that's the problem. Sadly, there isn't much cocoa in most chocolate. To profit from cocoa's health benefits, we'd better make sure we get it without the filler.

Fortunately, this has become more possible than ever before, because we are in the midst of a chocolate revolution in the United States. Just as Americans have learned to appreciate wine beyond the sticky-sweet limits of Gallo Burgundy, just as we've begun taking our coffee strong and dark, we're beginning to see the essence of chocolate beyond the wall of Hershey's Kisses. Dark chocolate—once relegated to the weird thing European visitors brought with them—is now the focus of a culinary awakening.

Walk into any supermarket these days and you will find

a range of chocolate bars to suit every palate. More and more artisanal chocolate makers are appearing on the world scene, and even the United States got its first new chocolate factory in fifty years when Scharffen Berger Chocolates opened in San Francisco in 1996. Many of these new chocolate bars proudly display the cocoa content right on them: 50, 60, even 70 percent (compared with a typical milk chocolate bar at 10 percent). Obviously, the more cocoa, the less room for fillers and additives, and the more health benefits. Baking trends, too, now favor the flourless chocolate torte or the intense, semisweet mousse over the wimpy cakes of years past. Clearly, the time is ripe for Americans to embrace chocolate as a serious food.

To do that, however, we're going to have to get over our guilt. Guilt and chocolate go hand in hand. Studies show chocolate to be far and away the most-craved food in existence, yet after indulging in it, many people feel guilty. Is it because they feel the chocolate is really so bad for them, or does it go deeper than that? America was founded by the Puritans, and a residual streak of Calvinist denial still runs through us. If being virtuous involves denying ourselves the things we most crave, and if chocolate is at the top of that craving list, then no wonder a lot of psychological baggage gets dragged into eating it.

Some of this guilt has manifested in a long list of evils attributed to chocolate, generally with flimsy evidence. As every teenage chocoholic knows, acne tops the list. Yet study after study has shown no connection between acne and chocolate (or any other food, for that matter). Migraines are another biggie disproved by research. Allergies? Hyperactivity? Nope. No evidence.

Believe it or not, chocolate even seems to be cleared of all charges in its indictment as a cavity-causer. Sugars are the raw material used by bacteria to make acid to drill holes in enamel, but the tannins in chocolate actually prevent the bacteria from sticking to teeth. So chocolate is probably the least likely type of sweet to cause cavities.

Then there is that other long-standing myth about chocolate. The reason Montezuma consumed fifty cups a day of the stuff, and Casanova couldn't get enough. The reason we soften up our sweethearts with it on Valentine's Day. Is chocolate an aphrodisiac? Not unless you want it to be, in which case, yes, it works quite well. Chocolate does, however, have an undeniable impact on mood. But because it is an extremely complex food, with more than 400 chemicals percolating away in it, we can only point to some likely causes.

Chocolate does contain caffeine, though in much lower levels than most of us think. A typical chocolate bar has about 10 mg of caffeine in it, compared to 135 mg in a cup of coffee. Other chemicals in chocolate are known mood-lifters, and one is almost identical to the THC found in marijuana. Likely, all these chemicals, and many others we haven't yet identified, combine to make chocolate a nice, mellow "feel-good" cocktail.

A feel-good cocktail that prevents heart disease, cancer, and cavities, and one that even tastes divine. Could it get any better? The answer is yes. For the past few years, cacao has again been raised sustainably in South and Central America, just as it was for millennia. This is an important consideration when choosing your chocolate, because by making the right choices you can support a return to sound agricultural and social practices—even as you're indulging yourself.

In the following chapters you'll learn a little history about this food that has had such a tremendous influence on both New World and Old, and you'll explore the amazing and unlikely process by which cacao beans are transformed into deep, rich chocolate. You'll see just how chocolate's positive effects on the heart and brain work, and I'll dismiss the myths about chocolate health problems once and for all. Along the way I'll foray into the basics of diet, for many of our assumptions about healthy eating have been overturned recently, and chocolate has a place in that. You'll discover who makes the most delicious, healthiest chocolate in the world, and I'll tell you where to get the good stuff.

The only requirement for you on this adventure is that you eat some quality chocolate while you read. Something dark, luscious, and brimming with the fruity, tantalizing hints of the rainforest where the beans were grown. Ready? Got your stash at hand? Here we go.

–1–

A Brief History of Chocolate

*F*or 95 percent of its three-thousand-year history, chocolate has been a drink and a health food. Both solid eating chocolate and the idea that chocolate is bad for you are twentieth-century inventions. The ancient Maya, whom we have to thank for perfecting chocolate culture, would have been quite skeptical of both notions.

But chocolate drinking predates the Maya by at least a thousand years. The Olmec, the Maya ancestors who thrived in Mesoamerica around 1000 B.C., had a sophisticated culture that included the carving of brilliant stone sculptures and the domestication of the basic New World food crops: maize, beans, squash, and chili peppers. They certainly must have farmed cacao as well, for the tree was native to the region and the sweet pulp of cacao pods would have been a draw from the time *Homo sapiens* first entered the New World. We have the Olmec to thank for the word *kakawa,* which the Maya transformed into *cacao,* the word we use to this day for the plant.

The Maya flourished throughout the first millennium A.D., and cacao flourished with them. Thanks to the Maya's own records, as well as the accounts of the Spanish conquistadors who encountered them in the sixteenth century, we know that the Maya had in place almost all of the advances in chocolate-making. We improved little on their techniques until the turn of the twentieth century (and even those "improvements" are questionable).

The Maya took cacao very seriously. They had a cacao god, and cacao was involved in many of their rituals. It was especially closely associated with blood, and sometimes played that role in their ceremonies. It was exchanged by the bride and groom during marriage ceremonies, much the way we use wedding rings. The Maya even had a type of baptism ceremony for children that involved anointing their heads with cacao water.

The Maya carefully tended groves of cacao, which grow best as understory trees and require constant water. They developed an elaborate trading system, most of it carried out by canoe, that stretched across all Mesoamerica (the area from Southern Mexico and Yucatan to Belize, Guatemala, and Honduras). Of all the products involved in this trade, cacao beans were the most important—so important, in fact, that they came to be used as currency. This makes it clear that cacao was highly valued, and that it was plentiful enough to go around and become the standard by which other products could be valued.

Maya artifacts depict cacao preparation much as it is carried out in Mesoamerica to this day. The beans were harvested, fermented, dried, ground into a paste, and then mixed with water and spices and drunk, usually hot. Of vital importance to properly prepared chocolate was the pouring of the liquid back and forth between two jars so that it frothed on top; the froth was considered the best part. The flavorings used in this original hot chocolate varied widely. Vanilla and chili peppers were extremely popular. Annatto, allspice, honey, maguey sap, sapote, and flower petals were also used. The chocolate was often mixed with corn and water to make a gruel. A similar corn-chocolate drink known as *pinole* is still common throughout Latin America. While we in the modern West tend to eat our grits or polenta in a thicker form, the Maya and many other ancient peoples, who were more concerned with conserving cooking fuel than we are, used these watery gruels as an easy way to get the day's nutrition in.

Historians are quick to point out that, as a sacred food, cacao in all its forms was not used to wash down tamales at breakfast. It was usually sipped alone, after dinner, much as we might break out a bottle of port. This is what the Spanish conquistadors observed, at least. And even the official Maya writings refer to chocolate only in conjunction with the upper classes—rulers, priests, warriors.

I'm not so sure. For starters, we know that at the very least cacao was used *in* the tamales—ceramic tamale platters have been found containing cacao residues. Likely it was used as a spice in a variety of dishes; the Maya were very sophisticated cooks. Historians may draw the wrong conclusions from examining the sacred texts of the Maya and the records of the Spanish, both of which focused on the behavior of the elite. This is like a future civilization attempting to learn about us and having nothing but Hollywood films to go on. They would conclude that 95 percent of the population smoked cigarettes. Everyday Maya wouldn't have had time, or inclination, to catalog their chocolate-drinking for history; they just had a cup and went on their way.

Common sense tells us that cacao was consumed in many different ways by most classes of Mesoamerican society, but that the majority of it went to the elite, and that this had more to do with economics than anything else. A sixteenth-century source reports that ten cacao beans could get you a rabbit or a prostitute, and one hundred could buy a slave. This tells us a couple of things. One, rabbits have gotten cheaper and prostitutes a lot pricier in the past five hundred years. Two, cacao was too valuable to simply swallow unless you had a lot of it on hand. Just as beluga caviar is considered a food of the upper classes—because who else is willing to waste fifty bucks on an appetizer?—the regular Maya probably couldn't afford to consume much cacao.

In the cities, at least. But don't believe books that tell you lower-class Maya consumed *no* chocolate, just because there is no record of it. Almost all surviving Maya records—as with most ancient civilizations—discuss the affairs of the rulers. From this, too many archaeologists seem to have concluded that not much worth recording was going on among the working class. But we know better. Do beluga fishermen reserve a little of the good stuff for themselves? Of course. Did Maya farmers and laborers pass every cacao bean on to the kings? Would you?

Any doubt that chocolate was enjoyed by regular Maya, at least in the outlying provinces, was dispelled by recent excavations at the El Salvadoran village of La Joya de Cerén. A volcano near the village erupted around 590 A.D., and the people just had time to flee before the village was buried in ash, like Pompeii, preserving everything as a snapshot in time. What this snapshot revealed, among other things, was a cacao tree in almost every yard. In this village, at least, cacao was not caviar. It was the mint patch out back.

Regardless of who got to drink it and who didn't, chocolate was valued so highly by the Maya that emperors were buried with jars of chocolate in their tombs. One such tomb featured an elaborate pottery screw-top jar with clear chocolate residues in it and the Maya hieroglyphics for cacao painted on the outside. Another obvious sign of cacao's value is the fact that, at another site, a jar was found filled with painstakingly carved *counterfeit* cacao beans, which were actually made of clay. Somebody went to a lot of trouble.

The first European to make contact with cacao was none other than Christopher Columbus. In 1502, on his last voyage to the New World, Columbus, along with his son Ferdinand, encountered a giant Maya dugout canoe off the Honduran Bay island of Guanaja. The canoe was more than one hundred feet long and was laden with goods to trade. Columbus did what he did best, immediately capturing the canoe and ransacking its supplies. Columbus and his men might not even have noticed the little dried beans the natives had with them, were it not that a few of the beans spilled on the ship as the natives were carrying goods aboard. The sight of these Maya scrambling for the beans (in the memorable words of Ferdinand) "as if an eye had fallen from their heads" alerted Columbus to the fact that these weren't your ordinary food staples. Still, Columbus had bigger fish to fry and couldn't bother himself with every bean that came along. He investigated cacao no further.

That job would fall to Hernán Cortés and his fellow conquistadors upon their arrival in Yucatan and Mexico in 1519. The Spaniards first made contact with the Maya in Yucatan, but it was the Aztec empire at Tenochtitlan—modern-day Mexico City—that captivated them. Here they found the gold and riches they so desperately craved, along with all the other wealth of a major empire. Tenochtitlan was one of the largest cities in the entire world at the time, and the Aztecs had conquered every other culture in Mesoamerica, including the Maya. From the Maya, they had inherited a taste for cacao. Though the tropical tree wouldn't grow anywhere near the cool highlands of Central Mexico, an elaborate trading system brought beans by the millions from the lowland rainforests of the Maya. Vast supplies of beans were shipped in tribute to the Aztecs from the conquered peoples of the south. A ruler of a medium-sized Aztec city went through millions of beans annually just to feed and pay his workers and soldiers, and the storehouses of the great Aztec king Montezuma were rumored to hold nearly a *billion* beans.

This impressed Cortés. The chocolate itself, however, didn't. The Aztecs drank their chocolate much as the Maya had, though they preferred it cold. Along with the rest of the Spaniards, Cortés found the bitter, strange substance undrinkable. And chocolate wasn't the only offender. The Spanish didn't have the most adventuresome palates, and they valued the native cuisine as poorly as they did other aspects of native culture. Chocolate, tortillas, and tamales were all considered only marginally better than starvation. A typical reaction was that of Girolamo Benzoni, who in his 1575 *History of the New World* called chocolate "more a drink for pigs than a drink for humanity."

As money, however, cacao was another story. In 1521, when the Spanish destroyed the Aztec empire and supplanted it as the rulers of the lands of Mesoamerica, they went right on using cacao as currency. In 1545 Mexico, one cacao bean could buy a tomato, an avocado, or a tamale. Three would get you a nice piece of fish. Though it is impossible to accurately compare prices across centuries, it seems that a cacao bean had a buying power in 1545 somewhat equivalent to a dollar today. Since it probably took at least ten beans to make a thin cup of chocolate, we can see why only the super-rich could afford to blow their cacao in such a manner. Astonishingly, this use of cacao as currency continued in parts of Mesoamerica into the nineteenth century.

The Spanish never did learn to like chocolate in the

native way, but as they got more comfortable with their new land, as they mingled and interbred with the locals, an early sort of fusion cuisine took place. Taking sugar from their newly established sugarcane plantations throughout the Caribbean islands, and mixing it with the cocoa of Mesoamerica, they discovered a drink that wasn't so bad. In fact, they quite liked it! The Creole population of the New World soon adopted the habit as well, and few have fought the sweetening trend since. So popular did chocolate become in Mexico that a seventeenth-century bishop in Chiapas was poisoned to death for refusing to allow his parishioners to bring their elaborate chocolate sets to mass.

It didn't take long for the colonists to bring chocolate back to Spain, where it immediately took hold—as a medicine. The Spanish did their best to keep the source of the drink a secret from their European rivals. And for a while they succeeded. When English buccaneers boarded a Spanish galleon in 1579, on its way back from the New World, they were terribly disappointed to find it loaded with what appeared to be "dried sheep's droppings." They burned the whole ship in frustration.

As mentioned at the beginning of this chapter, for most of its history chocolate has been thought of as health food, and it was in this guise that it conquered Europe. The Aztecs themselves believed that chocolate was healthy because it helped to cool down the body—a useful thing in the torrid tropics. Europe at the time was also dominated by a system of medicine based on the belief that health was a result of keeping the body balanced between hot and cold, dry and moist. If you tended to run hot and dry, you needed to take foods that were classified as cold and moist, and chocolate was considered just the thing.

In 1570, Francisco Hernández, royal physician to Philip II of Spain, recommended chocolate to cure fevers, cool the body in hot weather, and alleviate stomach pains. By the 1640s Roman physicians were recommending chocolate in the morning to soothe the stomach and aid in digestion, and the Cardinal of Lyon was drinking chocolate to "moderate the vapors of his spleen." A 1659 English advertisement for the newfangled chocolate drink claimed that it "cures and preserves the body of many diseases."

Chocolate swept seventeenth-century Europe as efficiently as the conquistadors had the New World. From its use as a medicine, it quickly spread to being drunk for pure pleasure as well. Taste certainly played a large role in this, but chocolate was also the first caffeinated beverage to reach Europe, beating tea and coffee by a few years. Of course, chocolate didn't pack the caffeine wallop of tea or coffee, but, as all decaf drinkers know, if you are used to no caffeine, a little can perk you right up.

As in the New World, chocolate in Europe was originally a drink of the aristocracy. A terrifically expensive import, it became associated with high-class entertaining. It was essential drinking in Louis XIV's court at Versailles. Europeans drank theirs hot and sweet, and mixed into it many of the New World spices, such as vanilla, but also quickly added cinnamon, from the Far East, and other exotic flavors. In Florence, Cosimo III de' Medici was famed for his jasmine chocolate, and wasn't above mixing in some ambergris and musk as well.

As we can see, demand for chocolate exploded after the 1500s. By the late seventeenth century, the traditional Maya groves in Mesoamerica couldn't possibly quench the world's thirst. And this is where chocolate first took its fall.

Until the seventeenth century, almost all cacao consumed in the world came from Mesoamerica. All this sublime cacao came from the same variety of tree—*criollo.* But faced with huge shortfalls in supply, caused by increased demand and by the devastation of the local population through diseases introduced by the Spanish, the Spanish needed to find another source. And they did.

In the South American rainforests, another variety of cacao tree was found. (Some scholars argue that South America was the original birthplace of the cacao tree, and that seeds were brought by humans to Mesoamerica.) This variety, known now as *forastero,* didn't have nearly the flavor of the *criollo* beans—it was more bitter and less aromatic—but it had some other distinct advantages. It produced many more pods, was less finicky in its growing conditions, and was less susceptible to disease. Faced with thundering demand, spiraling prices, and a new supply of cheap product, merchants did what merchants have always done: they jettisoned quality in favor of quantity. It didn't take the Spanish long to start vast groves in South America, with an endless supply of African slaves to tend them for free.

Did Europe's fine-palated aristocrats notice that their yummy chocolate was being replaced by coarser stuff? Far from it. Tastes had run so far toward the sweet end of the spectrum by that point that a few extra scoops of sugar covered up any bitterness that might have been detected. If Europeans had any remaining ability to detect the numerous and subtle flavor notes of *criollo* chocolate, the flooding of cheap and sweetened *forastero* onto the market killed it once and for all.

And this was just fine with chocolate producers. Nothing holds back an industry more than persnickety consumers who insist on fine flavors that come from a particular place. The great wine estates of France have their devoted fans who pay top dollar for the tiny amount of wine produced, but it is Gallo that makes the big bucks. To establish themselves as major chocolate purveyors with consistent product, the big nineteenth-century chocolate houses such as Nestlé, Cadbury, and Lindt had to have neutral-flavored cacao beans that could be mixed to deliver the same flavor in every batch.

Forastero was also one of the factors that finally brought chocolate to the masses. Huge supplies of high-yielding cacao trees brought the price down, and cutting the chocolate with more and more sugar—which came from the slave-driven Caribbean sugar plantations at much lower cost than cacao—brought the price down even further.

But it was the industrial revolution that truly democratized chocolate. In 1828, Coenraad Van Houten, a Dutchman, invented the process for making cocoa powder.

Then, by treating the powder with alkaline, Van Houten created "Dutch" chocolate that would easily mix with hot water. Cheap cocoa powder swept Europe and replaced the grainy, unmixable chocolate that had preceded it.

Even at this relatively late date, virtually all chocolate consumed in the world was in drink form. The 1850s changed all that. Joseph Fry, one of the largest names in English chocolate, discovered that, if you mixed cocoa powder and sugar with additional cocoa butter, instead of water, you could make a pliable paste that could be poured into molds and that would solidify as it cooled. Solid eating chocolate was born. Consumer reaction was predictable—people went crazy for the stuff. The addition of powdered milk to the mix—first accomplished in 1879 in Switzerland—made chocolate even more affordable and milder. It was now within reach of even the most meager pocketbooks and timid palates. By the turn of the twentieth century, drinking chocolate was a distant second to eating chocolate in popularity, and the gap has only grown since then.

It was Milton Hershey, of course, who finally made chocolate a ubiquitous presence in every grocery store. His large-scale industrial assembly lines and company town devoted to nothing but the making of chocolate were on a scale never imagined by his rivals. The famed Hershey's Kisses, for example, first introduced in 1907, are now churned out at the rate of 33 *million* per day.

But that still isn't enough to satisfy the world's hunger for chocolate. In 2003, 3 million metric tons of cacao were produced. The vast majority of this cacao is grown in West Africa. Mesoamerica, birthplace of chocolate, is no longer a central player in the chocolate story. Africa supplies 70 percent, with the Americas and Asia each supplying half of the remaining 30 percent.

With the abolition of slavery, cacao started to migrate from its ancestral home. The European powers could no longer bring Africans to the Americas to work the cacao plantations, so instead they brought the plantations to the Africans. And the cacao variety that made the trip was the high-yielding, disease-resistant, bitter *forastero*. Soon the vast plantations of West Africa dwarfed those in the Americas.

Cacao trees *hate* cold. They also hate dry. They need things warm and wet, so they can only grow within a strip ranging from 20 degrees north of the equator to 20 degrees below, and even there only in moist sections. After West Africa, cacao producers found another inviting location in Indonesia. Today, other countries growing cacao include India, Sri Lanka, and the South Pacific islands.

Virtually all of today's cacao (more than 90 percent) is *forastero*. *Criollo* is practically nonexistent. It isn't even the second-most popular variety. That title goes to *trinitario*, a hybrid of *forastero* and *criollo* first developed on the Caribbean island of Trinidad after a blight in 1727 wiped out the *criollo* groves there. The growers found that *trinitario* combined many of the best qualities of both its parents. It resisted disease and produced like a *forastero*, yet it tasted more like a *criollo*. Why didn't *trinitario* sweep the world instead of *forastero*? Perhaps *forastero* just had too much of a head start—or perhaps growers just couldn't be bothered with something so trivial as flavor.

But, like a good Hollywood film, this story has a last-minute reversal of fortune. *Criollo,* seemingly on its last legs and doomed to oblivion, has been rediscovered at the last minute, thanks to our exploding interest in taste, authenticity, and origin. Bucking a three-hundred-year trend, and following in the wake of similar awakenings in the worlds of wine, cheese, coffee, and tea, suddenly everybody wants single-origin chocolates exhibiting unique characteristics. And this means *criollo* (and *trinitario*). I'll discuss this more in the Resources section. For now, suffice it to say that high-end chocolate companies are scrambling to tie up the remaining handful of *criollo* and *trinitario* producers (mostly confined to the Caribbean and Venezuela), and this is a very good thing for the future of chocolate.

-2-

From Bean to Bonbon

*I*f presented with a cacao pod and asked to pick the edible part of it, my money would not have been on the seeds. Cacao seeds have "inedible" written all over them, and whoever first saw the culinary potential in the hard, bitter seeds was either a terrific visionary or terribly desperate. Probably both.

Cacao pods are the size and shape of a slightly deflated football and contain thirty to forty seeds each. The almond-sized seeds—known as *beans,* but, like coffee beans, not true beans—are encased in a sticky, white, yogurtlike pulp. The pulp is sweet, tart, and delicious. It's what I would eat if handed a cacao pod, and indigenous people have done just that for thousands of years. Certainly when the cacao plant was planning its reproductive future, the pulp is what it banked on.

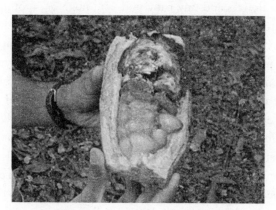

Mmm . . . a long way from dessert.

But along came humans, who, given the time and resources, will try to eat anything. The mango was a no-brainer, but the oyster? The caper? The artichoke? These took some outside-the-box thinking.

So, too, cacao. The path from cacao bean to finished chocolate is a long and surprising one, good to know about for its own sake, but which also may help us to appreciate even more that wonderful flavor we take for granted. It may also enlighten us to the difference in quality between various chocolates, so we'll know what to look for.

A good cacao tree can produce two thousand pods a year, and, unlike the temperate fruit trees most Americans are used to, those pods appear throughout the year. On a cacao tree you will see, growing straight out of the trunk, cacao flowers and tiny baby pods and huge one-pounders all growing side-by-side. For this reason, among others, cacao pods must be harvested by hand, carefully, so that the ripe pods can be taken without disturbing the still-growing ones. Many families in third-world countries all around the equator have harvested cacao for generations, and it is to their skill that we owe our enjoyment of chocolate.

After being cut from the trees with machetes or, for the higher pods, poles with blades on the end, the pods are either cut open right under the tree, and the seeds and pulp scraped into baskets, or the pods are brought back to a central area and opened there. It takes skill to open a pod without damaging the seeds inside, and again, this is something for which no machine can substitute for the experienced human hand. A good worker can open 500 pods per hour.

At this stage the cacao seeds (known as beans) are whitish-pink (if from the *criollo* variety) or purple (if *forasteros*) and wouldn't remind you of chocolate at all, in color, texture, or flavor. If you were foolish enough to try to eat one, you would know what bitterness was. This isn't accidental; the cacao pod's beautiful design serves to entice monkeys and other tropical animals into taking the pods, because of the sweet pulp. But if the monkeys ate the beans as well as the pulp, all would be lost. So the monkeys take the pods with them, eat the pulp, and learn very quickly to avoid the beans, tossing them aside—where a new cacao tree can take root.

But we monkeys have figured out a way to get around bitterness. It's called fermentation, and it's the reason for the next step in the process. Fermentation is a chemical

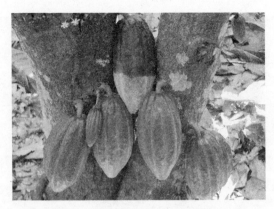

Cacao pods ripen throughout the year.

process, produced by the action of bacterial enzymes, where complex compounds are broken down into simple ones. In the case of cacao, the sugars in the pulp are broken down by enzymes into vinegar and other acids, and this step is essential to producing the chocolate flavor.

To encourage fermentation, workers heap the sticky, pulpy beans in large bins and cover them with banana leaves. Fermentation begins right away and causes the temperature to rise to around 120 degrees Fahrenheit. The pulp quickly turns to vinegar and melts away. Meanwhile, the bitter and astringent compounds in cacao are transformed into more palatable ones. The high temperature and acidity also kill the embryo inside the beans (the part that would become a seedling), which is necessary for the beans to start to take on chocolate flavors.

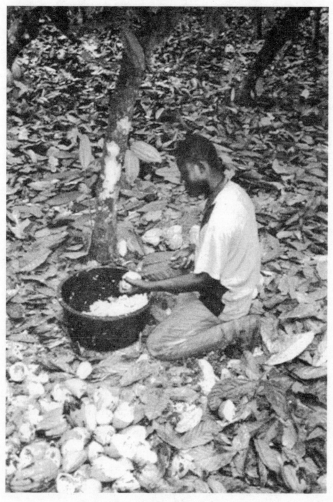

A cacao opener plying his trade.

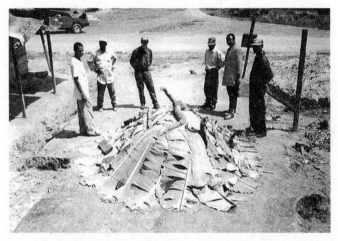

Cacao beans fermenting beneath banana leaves.

The length of fermentation depends on the variety of cacao used. *Criollos,* which aren't that bitter to begin with, only need a couple of days, while *forasteros* usually need six or more.

To stop the fermentation process, the beans are dried in the sun on long wooden trays and turned periodically. Other chemical changes necessary for flavor continue during this process. At night the trays are covered, or are rolled into sheds, to prevent moisture from settling on the beans. After several days, when the moisture content drops below 8 percent, the chemical changes cease. The beans have lost half their original weight at this point. They are now brown and ready to be shipped to the factory. (Unless, of course, the factory is right there *in* the rainforest; see the Grenada Chocolate Company in the Resources section.)

At the factory, the beans are roasted at about 230 degrees for at least twenty minutes. (Again, *criollos* need less time than *forasteros*.) As with coffee, the roasting deepens the flavor and darkens the beans. With coffee, an ultra-dark French roast style is only a good idea with inferior beans; truly aromatic coffee benefits from a lighter roast that won't cover up its intrinsic flavors with a burnt one. The same goes for wonderfully aromatic cacao.

We now have brittle, dark brown beans that start to look and smell like chocolate. But the dry, fibrous shells still need to be removed to get to the creamier beans inside. So they are rolled through a machine where they are lightly crushed—cracked, really—which allows the lightweight husks to be winnowed away by blown air. What's left are the cracked pieces of bean known as *nibs*. These nibs are the raw material of chocolate. (Some chocolate makers now offer bars laced with crunchy, crackly nibs; don't miss an opportunity to try one.)

The nibs are crushed in a mill, where they form a thick paste known as *cocoa liquor*. The word *liquor* is a bit misleading; there's nothing alcoholic about it, and it isn't really a liquid. Think instead of grainy, black-bean paste. This paste is about half cocoa butter and half cocoa solids.

And now we come to a fork in the road. What you do next with that grainy cocoa liquor depends on your final product.

Dark Chocolate

If you are making true chocolate, you need to change the viscosity and texture of your paste into something that will be smooth and moldable. This is accomplished in two ways: first, by beating the heck out of cocoa liquor with heavy machines; second, by adding extra cocoa butter (the natural fat of the cacao seeds) and, almost always, lecithin.

The machines get the first crack at the cocoa liquor. After being mixed with powdered sugar and any other flavors required for the particular product (vanilla is quite common), the liquor is passed through a refiner—steel rollers set less than 1/1000 of an inch apart. This ensures perfect smoothness, no lumps.

Then comes one of the secrets of modern chocolate: the conche. Named for its shell-like shape, the conche was invented in 1879 by the Swiss Rodolphe Lindt, founder of the Lindt chocolate empire. The cocoa liquor is poured into the shell of the conche, which acts like a giant dough mixer. A series of rollers plow through the mass and slosh it back and forth, from only a few hours for low-grade chocolate to as much as three days for the good stuff. Conching not only reduces the particle size of the cocoa and sugar crystals even further—improving the plasticity—but also triggers one final round of flavor changes.

But machinery alone can't transform cocoa liquor to chocolate. For that, we need extra fat, without which chocolate would be hard, brittle stuff. The fat of choice, of course, is cocoa butter, but lecithin is also needed. Lecithin is a flavorless vegetable fat, usually obtained from soy beans, and it is a much better emulsifier than cocoa butter. It helps give chocolate its velvety texture and unctuous feel. It is also far cheaper than cocoa butter, and therein lies a problem. Chocolate makers not concerned with flavor can improve their bottom lines by extracting the cocoa butter from their cocoa liquor, selling it to the cosmetics industry, where it is in high demand because it is an excellent fat for the skin, and using cheap lecithin to make up the difference. The resulting product has less depth of cocoa flavor, but that hardly matters, when sugar is what consumers of these cheap chocolates are really looking for.

It's worth noting that lecithin and sugar are far from the only ingredients with which chocolate has been cut during its history. The nineteenth century is rife with accounts of "doctored" chocolate. Common ingredients used to cut chocolate included flour made from rice, wheat, lentils, barley, peas, or potatoes, mutton fat, arrow root, and almond oil. The situation got so bad that the British medical journal *The Lancet* studied 70 samples of chocolate in 1950 and found that 39 of them had been colored with red brick dust! Today we needn't worry about any of that; by law, pure chocolate can only contain cocoa liquor, cocoa butter, sugar, lecithin, vanilla, and milk (if milk chocolate). And with sugar, lecithin, and milk among the cheapest available ingredients, there is little incentive for the unscrupulous to try to doctor chocolate any longer.

After cocoa butter and lecithin are added during the

conching process (which, thanks to friction, also heats the mass up), the mixture—which can now truly be called chocolate—is tempered as it cools. Tempering involves constant stirring, so that the crystals in the cocoa butter remain in suspension and don't form bonds that would result in blotchy, granular chocolate.

The final stage is to pour warm, liquid chocolate into molds, whether in the shape of bars, bunnies, or eggs, where it will fully cool and solidify. One of the beauties of cocoa butter is that it is one of the few substances that turns from solid to liquid at just below body temperature, meaning all it takes is a willing tongue to melt that chocolate. Of course, this quality also makes chocolate the bane of car seats and five-year-olds' pockets.

Milk Chocolate

The making of milk chocolate follows the same process as that of dark chocolate (or plain chocolate, as it is known in Britain), with one important difference: milk, either powdered or condensed, is added to the liquor before it is refined and conched. The creaminess and mild flavor of milk chocolate have triumphed over the "grown-up" taste of dark chocolate, but chocolate manufacturers may have had another reason for marketing their milk chocolate first: milk, like sugar, is far cheaper than cacao. The history of food in the twentieth century has involved a movement away from strong flavors of any kind and toward

extremely mild flavors that wouldn't offend anyone—
think of American beers, Wonder bread, and American
cheese. The reaction against this in the past two decades,
with a resurgence of interest in wine, beer, cheese, bread,
coffee, and now chocolate with distinctive flavor and per-
sonality, is a heartening development indeed.

Cocoa Powder

Like modern, satiny-smooth chocolate, cocoa powder
also owes its existence to the industrial revolution. But
whereas the Swiss were responsible for the most important breakthroughs in chocolate manufacture, it was the
previously mentioned Dutchman, Coenraad Van Houten,
who created the first cocoa powder.

After cocoa nibs are ground, the resulting cocoa liquor
is about half solids and half cocoa butter. Van Houten first
seized upon the idea of submitting the liquor to intense
pressure—up to 6,000 pounds per square inch—in huge
hydraulic presses, to squeeze out about half of the cocoa
butter. There were two huge advantages to this: first, the
pure cocoa butter has always claimed a premium price in
the food, pharmaceutical, and cosmetics industries; and
second, the resulting low-fat "press cake" could be pulver-
ized into a powder with numerous utilitarian possibilities.
While cocoa powder lacks the flavor of true chocolate, it
is much more versatile. On the industrial scale, lightweight and stable cocoa powder was much easier to work

into mass-produced goods, whether ice cream or fudge.

On the consumer scale, instead of making hot chocolate by scraping bits of chocolate off a block of solid chocolate and melting it in water or milk, people could now simply mix the powder in water with a minimum of fuss. The only problem is that cocoa powder doesn't easily mix with water. It tends to clump together. Van Houten solved this dilemma by treating the powder with an alkali. While this made it easier to mix, it also lightened the flavor and darkened the color. A problem? Not at all. Many people found they preferred the lighter flavor of this "Dutch" cocoa, and to this day Dutch cocoa—probably because of the association Americans have between continental Europe and quality—is sometimes erroneously sought out as a superior product.

The Proof Is in the Pudding

So there you have it, the long journey from bean to bonbon. As we've seen, a dizzying number of factors go into the final quality of chocolate. Everything from cacao variety to processing techniques and especially mix of ingredients helps determine how chocolate affects your palate and your arteries. And now that you've had an hors d'oeuvre of history and an appetizer of process, it's time for the main course: the amazing health properties of your favorite confection.

-3-

Chocolate *Is* Health Food

*O*kay, now it is time to convince you. Chocolate really is good for you. Before you say, "Yeah, right," remember that "Yeah, right" is what we said when they first told us red wine was good for us. "Yeah, right" is what we said when they told us olive oil was good for us. We still carry old assumptions—perhaps from many decades of mushy vegetables in the United States, or from well-meaning mothers—that has us convinced of a split in the food world: there are foods that are good for us, and foods that taste good, and rarely do the two sides mix. Broccoli, spinach, whole-wheat bread: good for us, taste bad. Wine, nuts, chocolate: bad for us, taste good.

Thankfully, just as we are learning how delicious broccoli and spinach can be, just as we now take it for granted that moderate wine drinking is good for our hearts, we will soon see it as self-evident that chocolate is good for us. But that time is still a bit off, so we'd better go through the evidence anyway.

Members of the jury, I now call antioxidants to the stand.

What Are Antioxidants?

Although everyone has heard of antioxidants, most people have only a hazy conception of what they are. These compounds, found in fruits and vegetables, help prevent scores of diseases—everything from heart disease and cancer to stroke, Alzheimer's disease, rheumatoid arthritis, cataracts, and the general effects of aging. Antioxidants are what make carrots orange and tomatoes red. Some antioxidants have been well known for years, such as vitamin C and vitamin E; others have been recognized only recently.

Among the most noteworthy antioxidants are polyphenols, the compounds in red wine and green tea that are so good for our blood vessels. You don't need a lab to confirm the presence of polyphenols in red wine and tea; just use your tongue. That astringency and hint of bitterness comes from the polyphenols. Can you think of any other foods that produce astringency and bitterness on the tongue? That's right: chocolate.

If bitterness is not the first word that comes to mind when you think of chocolate, think instead of cocoa powder or baking chocolate. That bitterness is the key, because it marks the sign of certain concentrated polyphenol antioxidants. And I mean concentrated: a bar of dark

Top Antioxidant Foods

	ORAC* units per 100 g
Dark Chocolate	13,120
Milk Chocolate	6,740
Prunes	5,770
Raisins	2,830
Blueberries	2,400
Blackberries	2,036
Kale	1,770
Strawberries	1,540
Spinach	1,260
Raspberries	1,220
Brussels Sprouts	980
Plums	949
Alfalfa Sprouts	930
Broccoli Florets	890
Oranges	750
Red Grapes	739
Red Bell Pepper	710
Cherries	670
Onions	450
Corn	400
Eggplant	390

*ORAC (Oxygen Radical Absorbance Capacity) is a measure of the ability of foods to subdue harmful oxygen free radicals that can damage our bodies.
Source: Data from the U.S. Department of Agriculture and the Journal of the American Chemical Society.

chocolate has twice the antioxidant content of a glass of red wine and seven times that of green tea. What about fruits and vegetables? They don't even come close. Oranges have 750 antioxidant units per 100 grams, kale 1,770. Blueberries, poster-children of the antioxidant world, have 2,400. And dark chocolate? More than 13,000.

"Chocolate just stands out," says Joe Vinson of the University of Scranton, Pennsylvania. "It's much higher than anything else." Other studies have shown that one good-quality dark chocolate bar can have more polyphenols than two whole days' worth of fruits and vegetables.

If it seems amazing that a confection could blow away all these healthy fruits and vegetables, remind yourself that chocolate is made from the seeds of a fruit. Easten in fairly pure form, chocolate fits perfectly into a healthy, all-natural diet.

How Antioxidants Work

What is so magical about antioxidants? How can they help prevent such a wide range of diseases? To understand, we need to look a little closer at the basic workings of the body.

When you hear the term *free radical,* do you picture an aging hippie living in Berkeley? If so, you may be alarmed to learn that legions of free radicals are coursing through your body right now. Free radicals are molecules gone bad: they have had one of their electrons knocked off, or have had an extra electron forced upon them, so they have a charge. But (as we all remember from chemistry class) molecules don't want a charge, they want to be neutral, so free radicals search their environment for a place to unload their extra electron, if they have too many, or steal an electron if they are one short.

Of course, the molecule victimized by the original free radical now has a charge of its own. So what does it do? It turns around and does the same thing to its neighbor. A chain reaction occurs that continues until something else comes along to intervene.

Now picture a free radical in your body. If it steals an electron from one of your cells, you then have a chain reaction of radical cells in your body. If it attacks your DNA, so much the worse. Cells don't respond well to having their molecular structure altered. Cancer is just one of many diseases resulting from this. Blame free radicals for everything from wrinkled skin to memory loss, immune system deterioration, and arthritis. Blame free radicals for much of what we chalk up to "aging."

One of the most common diseases linked to free radicals is atherosclerosis—hardening of the arteries. Cholesterol and fatty substances build up on the interior walls of arteries, slowly blocking the flow of blood. Complete blockage of blood flow can result in a heart attack or stroke. The problem is enormous: cardiovascular disease is the number-one killer of Americans, responsible for 39 percent of the deaths in this country, with cancer coming in a distant second at 23 percent.

Free radicals cause atherosclerosis by damaging the

endothelium—the inner wall of the artery. Normally this wall is perfectly smooth, allowing molecules in the blood to pass by unhindered. But by scavenging electron fragments from the wall, free radicals "scuff up" the wall. (Think of a Teflon frying pan when it's new, and then after it has been hacked at with a spatula for a year: foods start to stick. The same thing happens in your arteries.) Fatty substances get caught by the no-longer-smooth surfaces, and as they stick, they start to trap other passersby. Soon, this plaque grows into a major obstruction. Free radicals make the situation even worse by "scuffing" the cholesterol molecules in the bloodstream, too, making them more likely to latch on to each other and to arterial walls.

Now the bad news: you have scads of free radicals in your body, and there is no way to prevent this. Free radicals are a natural by-product of basic bodily processes such as respiration and digestion. However, they are also increased by a number of far less natural processes: radiation, smoking, consumption of alcohol, preservatives, and chlorinated drinking water, and exposure to pollution and even sunlight. So it behooves us to minimize our exposure as much as possible, and to do everything we can to neutralize the free radicals within us. The body's immune system eliminates as many free radicals as it can, but it can't possibly get them all. The average DNA receives 10,000 "hits" from free radicals per *day*. The body needs all the help it can get.

Enter the antioxidants. Antioxidants neutralize free radicals in several ways. The polyphenol antioxidants in chocolate are molecules composed of a ring of six carbon atoms. Some of the bonds between the carbon atoms are double bonds, but a single bond between carbon atoms is all that's necessary for the molecule to hold together, so polyphenols can easily "shuffle" their bonds to have one free to latch onto a charged particle that comes along— like a free radical. They then carry the free radical out of the body with them when they are excreted through normal processes.

As you can see, your body needs a constant supply of polyphenols and other antioxidants to continuously eliminate free radicals from the body. Chocolate is one of the best places to get this supply.

The Panama Paradox

Antioxidants may not be the only heart-healthy compounds in chocolate. You've heard of the French Paradox, right? The fact that the French eat more saturated fat than do Americans but have much lower rates of heart disease? The paradox is that saturated fat is supposed to clog the arteries. The answer? The polyphenols in all that red wine the French drink help to protect their arteries against the damaging effects of all that fat.

Now, let's talk about the Panama Paradox. On a group of islands off the coast of Panama dwell the Kuna people. This indigenous group eats a traditional diet high in salt, yet they have extremely low blood pressure. As did their Central

American ancestors, the Kuna drink about five cups of chocolate a day. Could the chocolate be responsible for their low blood pressure? It seemed possible, because blood pressure rose in the Kuna who moved to urban Panama City and stopped consuming their traditional diet.

To test chocolate's role in this, Norman Hollenberg, professor of medicine at Harvard University, fed Boston volunteers either typical commercial milk chocolate or dark chocolate bars. Those who consumed the dark chocolate at levels equivalent to the cocoa intake of the Kuna islanders showed the same high levels of nitric oxide in their blood. This is worth noting because nitric oxide is responsible for relaxing and dilating blood vessels, which lowers blood pressure and allows more blood to pass through them unimpeded.

Tasty Aspirin?

The nitric oxide effect of chocolate may also be behind the evidence that chocolate seems to help prevent blood platelets from clumping and forming clots. By blocking the flow of blood, clots cause heart attacks and strokes. Carl Keen, chairman of the nutrition department at the University of California-Davis, found that a drink containing 25 grams of semisweet chocolate had the same thinning effect on blood platelets as did an 81-milligram dose of aspirin. So it's your choice: an after-dinner aspirin, or a couple squares of dark chocolate?

Chocolate Studies

All this is great in theory, but what about putting it to the test? Sure, polyphenols prevent heart disease, stroke, and other diseases, and cocoa is loaded with polyphenols, but has cocoa been proven to have health benefits? Let's look at the research.

A study at Pennsylvania State University had volunteers eat 22 grams of cocoa powder and 16 grams of dark chocolate in their daily diets. The volunteers had much improved cholesterol ratios, with more of the good HDL cholesterol and less of the bad LDL cholesterol. Most interesting, and surely related to chocolate's antioxidant effect, the LDL cholesterol that did exist seemed to be more resistant to oxidation—the process where it is "scuffed up" by free radicals and becomes more sticky. A similar study in 1996 found that subjects' LDL cholesterol was much more resistant to oxidation two hours after they had eaten 35 grams of cocoa powder. Another study conducted on cocoa-fed rabbits found the same effect.

I hesitate to tell you about this next study. The results sound so over-the-top that they can only make people look at you funny when you tell them. But you should probably tell them anyway. Two researchers at the Harvard School of Public Health studied 7,800 Harvard alumni and found that those who ate chocolate and other candy 1 to 3 times per month lived, on average, a year longer than those who never ate candy. Those who pounded candy—at least 3 times per week—didn't live quite as long, but still were 16 percent less likely to die over the period of the study than the candy abstainers. Don't take this as a license to inhale every ice cream cone you see—remember, it's best to up your chocolate intake without increasing sugar consumption—but now and then, it's probably a healthy thing to let the good times roll.

Other Antioxidant Studies

Though the studies have not yet been undertaken to prove it, there are strong reasons to believe that chocolate can help protect you against many other illnesses besides cardiovascular disease as well. We know that free radicals are associated with many of the diseases that are the scourge of modern society—everything from cancer and Alzheimer's disease to rheumatoid arthritis and cataracts. We know that antioxidants cleanse the body of free radicals. And we know that chocolate is abundant in flavonoids, some of the most potent polyphenol antioxidants known (100 times more potent than vitamin C). So, although studies using chocolate are just beginning, let's examine some of the thousands of studies done on antioxidants in general, and flavonoid-rich foods in particular, and see what we can infer about chocolate.

Cardiovascular Disease
The evidence linking antioxidants to reduced cardiovascular disease is overwhelming. A study at Brigham and

Women's Hospital in Boston of 1,800 nurses with histories of coronary problems found that women who consumed high amounts of antioxidant-rich foods had a 33 percent lower risk of heart attack and a 71 percent lower risk of stroke compared to women who ate few foods containing antioxidants.

Much of the best evidence involves consumption of red wine, which, as we've discussed, contains the same flavonoids (a subgroup of polyphenols) as chocolate. Huge studies, such as the American Cancer Society Study of 276,802 people and the Nurse's Health Study of 87,526 women, all show a 20 to 40 percent decrease in coronary heart disease among moderate drinkers, compared to nondrinkers. The most recent, most conclusive study—a Harvard School of Public Health study of 38,000 men over twelve years—also found a 30 to 35 percent lower risk of heart attack in those who consumed alcohol, especially those who consumed it regularly.

For surveying health studies, tea is probably an even better stand-in for chocolate than is red wine. Tea and chocolate contain the same flavonoids as red wine, though chocolate has the flavonoids in even greater concentrations. Tea and chocolate also both contain caffeine, but no alcohol. Unlike chocolate, tea has been extensively studied over the past ten years to determine its potential as a health food. Numerous studies have confirmed its power to prevent heart disease, cancer, and many other diseases, and there is overwhelming evidence that the flavonoids are responsible. It seems likely that chocolate's powers of health prevention are in line with those of tea.

One tea study at Beth Israel Deaconess Medical Center of people recovering from heart attacks found that, in the three and a half years following their heart attacks, heavy tea drinkers (those who drank more than two cups per day) had a 44 percent lower death rate than did non-tea-drinkers, while moderate tea drinkers had a 28 percent lower rate. Other recent studies with tea confirmed that it improves the ability of blood vessels to dilate and that it has an anticlotting effect. As with chocolate, flavonoids are believed to be the compounds responsible for this effect.

In Japan, people who drank at least three cups of tea per day had an 11 percent lower risk of heart attack than people who drank less tea than that. Japanese who drank 5 to 10 cups per day live longer than those who don't.

Another recent study at the USDA had volunteers drink five cups of tea-flavored water for three weeks, followed by five cups a day of real tea for the same period. The tea drinking resulted in a 10 percent reduction in bad LDL cholesterol rates, but no change in good HDL cholesterol.

Cancer

A study at the University of Hawaii's Cancer Research Center found that those who ate the most flavonoids in their diet had a 40 to 50 percent reduced rate of lung cancer. A study of 6,000 Italian citizens found that those who ate at least ten different varieties of vegetables per week were 30 percent less likely to develop colorectal cancer than those who ate less than seven varieties per week. The antioxidants in vegetables are the suspected reason. And in the most thorough study done to date, a twenty-four-year

Finnish study of 10,000 people, those who consumed the most flavonoids were 20 percent less likely to develop any form of cancer than those who consumed the fewest.

Studies on mice have shown that the flavonoids in tea protect against skin tumors, lung cancer, and digestive cancer. In addition, lab cellular studies demonstrated that tea flavonoids inhibited the reproduction of human leukemia and lung carcinoma cells. A team at Georgetown University is currently working on isolating the flavonoids in chocolate and testing them as an anticancer drug.

At the Arizona Cancer Center, 140 smokers were given either green tea, black tea, or water for four months to study the effect on a particular free radical known to cause DNA damage. The green-tea drinkers had 25 percent fewer of the free radicals, while there was no change in the black-tea drinkers. This makes sense, since some of the flavonoids in tea are destroyed in the process by which black tea is made.

Alzheimer's Disease

The brain lesions characteristic of Alzheimer's disease are caused by free radicals scavenging their way through brain tissue. Not surprisingly, many studies have established links between consumption of antioxidant-rich foods and prevention of Alzheimer's. For example, a recent study of 815 Chicago residents over age 65, published in the *Journal of the American Medical Association,* showed that those who consumed the most vitamin E foods were 70 percent less likely to develop Alzheimer's than those who consumed the least. Another study of 5,400 Dutch residents found that those who consumed the most vitamin C were 18 percent less likely to develop Alzheimer's than those who consumed the least.

Vitamins C and E are different types of antioxidants than the flavonoids found in chocolate. However, a 2002 study of 1,700 Danes found that those who drank at least one glass of red wine per week were much less likely to develop Alzheimer's than those who never drank red wine. No benefit was found from drinking other types of alcohol, indicating that the flavonoids in red wine are likely responsible. Similarly, the PAQUIN study, one of the most significant Alzheimer's studies undertaken, showed that those who consume the most flavonoids in their diet had only half the usual incidence of Alzheimer's.

Interestingly, proanthocyanidin, one of the flavonoids in chocolate, is one of the few compounds that can cross the blood-brain barrier, where it can directly work its protective effects on brain tissue.

Arthritis

Rheumatoid arthritis tortures the lives of more than two million people in the United States. But a recent study of mice showed that the polyphenols in green tea may significantly reduce one's risk of getting the disease. In the study, 36 mice were injected with collagen, which induces arthritis in rodents. Half the mice were fed the human equivalent of four cups of green tea per day. Of the 18 who didn't receive the green tea, 17 developed arthritis. Of the 18 who did receive the green tea, only 8 developed arthritis, and even in those mice it was a milder form of the disease. Scientists believe it is the anti-inflammatory power of tea's polyphenols that achieves the effect. Arthritis is partially caused by free radicals attacking the joint membranes and lubricants, leading to inflammation, so neutralizing the free radicals prevents the inflammation from forming in the first place.

Proanthocyanidin, the antioxidant in chocolate that may protect against Alzheimer's, may also reduce arthritis symptoms. Proanthocyanidin, which is also found in red wine, blocks the formation of enzymes in the body that cause inflammation.

Asthma and Allergies

For the same reasons that proanthocyanidin can reduce inflammation in arthritis sufferers, it can also reduce symptoms of asthma and allergies. Both conditions are caused by the body's immune system attacking invaders with histamines. Proanthocyanidins act as antihistamines, blocking the body's release of histamines.

Cough Suppressant

While all the studies mentioned so far involve chocolate's antioxidant compounds, researchers at the National Heart and Lung Institute in London are exploring a completely different healing aspect of chocolate. They tested the cough-relieving ability of theobromine, a stimulant found in chocolate, against codeine, the traditional ingredient in cough medicines. Theobromine was more effective. As the

British newspaper *The Express* put it, "A bar of chocolate works better than a spoonful of medicine in treating a cough." The researchers are now trying to determine whether theobromine works by suppressing the cough itself or by clearing mucus from the lungs.

The Big Picture

Chocolate reduces your risk of heart disease by what percent? Antioxidants have what effect on cancer? Too much research can be difficult to take in. So don't bother trying to keep it all in your head—it's too stressful, among other things, and stress isn't good for your blood pressure! You don't need to leave this chapter as a walking, talking chocolate encyclopedia; just know that the evidence for chocolate is there, and that it's rigorous. Scientists will be debating for years *how* good chocolate is for you; they no longer seriously question *whether* it's good for you. Forget the figures; just eat your chocolate, and relax.

– 4 –

What's in Chocolate?

*W*hen people knock chocolate, they usually take one of two lines of attack: either "chocolate is full of bad fat" or "chocolate is full of sugar." Both of these positions display a lack of knowledge about chocolate and nutrition in general. In this chapter, we'll set the facts straight and learn just what *is* in that brownie, and whether you need to worry about it.

The Skinny on Fat

Back in the 1980s, nutritionists thought they had it all figured out. Fat, they declared, was the enemy. Stay away from fat and cholesterol, stick to protein and carbohydrates, and you will be skinny, happy, and long-lived.

And we listened. Low-fat became all the rage. Out went the olive oil from salad dressings; in went lots of sugar to make up for the tastelessness of watery dressings. Great piles of fat-free pasta became the entrée du jour.

But a funny thing happened on the way to the scale. While our *fat intake* went down, we got *fatter.* The percentage of fat in the American diet began going down in the 1980s and has been declining ever since, but an obesity epidemic began in the United States *at the exact same time.* Today obesity is a larger problem than ever before. We have three times as many obese children as we had in the 1980s.

Meanwhile, the nutritionists continued to change their tune. After trying to stick to their story that all fat was evil, period, despite strong evidence to the contrary, in the late 1980s they admitted that maybe certain fats were good for you. Like olive oil—which turned out to lower your cholesterol level. Soon they came up with a new consensus: all fat still made you fat, but now fat was divided into three types: monounsaturated fat, such as olive oil; polyunsaturated fat, such as corn oil, soybean oil, and margarine; and saturated fat, such as butter, animal fat, coconut oil, and cocoa butter. The monounsaturated fats kept your heart and blood vessels healthy, the polyunsaturated fats had a neutral effect, and the saturated fats killed you quick: a stick of butter was a heart attack on a plate.

Trouble was, this still didn't seem to jibe with the evidence. People cut out the beef, butter, and eggs and ate margarine on their potatoes, yet obesity, diabetes, and cardiovascular disease continued to explode.

Now scientists are learning that it is much more complicated than the simple categories they created. While olive oil clearly has strong benefits for the heart and arteries, the polyunsaturated fats, such as corn oil, may be the real problem—especially when made into *trans* fats, which happens when vegetable oils are turned from liquids into solids, as they are in margarine and the numerous processed foods on supermarket shelves such as cookies, crackers, and baked goods. Trans fats are also created during deep frying.

Surprisingly, saturated fats are now beginning to lose their reputation as the bad guys. Most studies show a weak link at best between saturated fat intake and disease. Indigenous tribes such as the Masai and Eskimo consume diets extraordinarily high in saturated fat (beef, milk, and blood for the Masai; blubber for the Eskimo), yet cardiovascular disease is unknown to them—until they diverge from their traditional diet.

What is becoming more and more evident is that not all saturated fats are alike; in fact, the health impact of different saturated fats is so varied that it makes little sense to include them all in the same category.

Chocolate is a prime example of this. Cocoa butter—the fat that occurs naturally in cacao beans—has a fair amount of fat in it, a lot of it saturated. A typical dark chocolate bar will have about 11 grams of fat, 7 of which are saturated, so people have long assumed that this made it "bad" for you. But if we look a little deeper, we discover the real story. The 4 grams of unsaturated fat are composed of oleic acid, the same fatty acid that makes olive oil good for you. Oleic acid raises your good HDL cholesterol level and lowers your bad LDL cholesterol. Of the saturated fat, more than half is composed of stearic acid, a fatty acid that is converted by the liver to oleic acid. That's right, the same stuff as olive oil.

Because evidence points to stearic acid being given a bad rap, studies are beginning to focus on it. One such study fed men three different diets for three weeks each: the first was high in oleic acid, the second in stearic acid, and the third in palmitic acid (the dominant fatty acid in beef, pork, and dairy). Palmitic acid is believed to be the primary culprit in raising cholesterol levels and contributing to atherosclerosis. Compared to the high-palmitic-acid diet, the high-oleic-acid diet reduced cholesterol levels by 10 percent, but the high-stearic-acid diet reduced cholesterol levels by 14 percent. Many other studies have shown that stearic acid does not raise cholesterol levels at all.

What about chocolate itself? While stearic and oleic acids are its dominant fatty acids, 25 percent of its fat is palmitic acid, the not-so-good stuff. But the high levels of good fats seem to counteract the potential negative effect of the bad fat. Back in the 1960s, two important studies were already showing no effect on cholesterol from diets high in cocoa butter. More recently, researchers at Pennsylvania State University fed volunteers 10 ounces of milk chocolate per day, raising the subjects' percentage of calories from saturated fat from 14 to 20. There was no effect on cholesterol. When the same test was done using butter instead of chocolate to supply the saturated fat, cholesterol rates went up.

The same researchers also had volunteers consume a diet recommended by the American Heart Association, but then substituted a bar of milk chocolate for a high-carb snack in the diet. This increased fat content in the diet by 4 percent and reduced carbohydrate content accordingly. The result? No change in bad LDL cholesterol, but an increase in good HDL cholesterol, meaning less chance of stroke and heart disease. No doubt the numbers would have been even better if dark chocolate had been used instead of milk chocolate.

What's the upshot of all this? While it would be a stretch to claim that the fat in chocolate is good for your heart, it clearly isn't bad for it, either. It isn't as good for you as olive oil fat, but it's better than beef, pork, or dairy fat, and much better than trans fats. And if indulging in chocolate keeps you from reaching for truly unhealthy foods—such as ice cream, French fries, or doughnuts—then it is doing you a favor indeed.

Chocolate Nutrients

But enough about fat. There's more to chocolate than that. A typical chocolate bar contains a number of nutrients that make it look suspiciously like . . . food. A glance at the USDA's own information on dark chocolate reveals that a bar contains a couple of grams each of protein and fiber, and significant amounts of iron, copper, zinc, phosphorus, and magnesium. The magnesium is particularly noteworthy, because magnesium regulates blood pressure and protects from heart disease, augmenting the abilities of

Nutrient Information of Dark Chocolate

Nutrient	Units	Value per 100 g	1 bar (1.55 oz) 44.00 g
Energy	kcal	479.00	210.76
Energy	kj	2004.00	881.76
Protein	g	4.20	1.85
Total Fat	g	30.00	13.20
Total Carbohydrate	g	63.10	27.76
Fiber	g	5.90	2.60
Sugars	g	56.90	25.04
Calcium, Ca	mg	32.00	14.08
Iron, Fe	mg	3.13	1.38
Magnesium, Mg	mg	115.00	50.60
Phosphorus, P	mg	132.00	58.08
Potassium, K	mg	365.00	160.60
Sodium, Na	mg	11.00	4.84
Zinc, Zn	mg	1.62	0.71
Copper, Cu	mg	0.70	0.31
Manganese, Mn	mg	0.80	0.35
Selenium, Se	mcg	3.10	1.36
Vitamin C	mg	0.00	0.00
Thiamine	mg	0.06	0.02
Riboflavin	mg	0.09	0.04
Niacin	mg	0.43	0.19
Pantothenic acid	mg	0.11	0.05
Vitamin B6	mg	0.034	0.02
Folate	mcg	3.00	1.32
Vitamin B12	mcg	0.00	0.00
Vitamin A	IU	21.00	9.24
Vitamin A, RE	mcg RE	2.00	0.88
Vitamin E	mg ATE	1.19	0.52
Fatty acids, saturated	g	17.75	7.81
Fatty acids, monounsaturated	g	9.97	4.39
Fatty acids, polyunsaturated	g	0.97	0.43
Cholesterol	mg	0.00	0.00
Caffeine	mg	62.00	27.28
Theobromine	mg	486.00	213.84

Source: USDA Nutrient Database for Standard Reference, Release 13 (November 1999)

chocolate's antioxidants to do these same things. In addition, magnesium improves the way carbohydrates are metabolized, making it easier for the body to deal with the sugar in chocolate.

Now, there is one nutrient on this list that you do need to watch out for, and it isn't the saturated fat. It's the sugar. Twenty-five grams of simple carbohydrates. The candy companies will tell you that sugar has a clean bill of health; that it hasn't been linked to any diseases or even obesity, that unless you're a diabetic, you needn't worry about sugar. So far, most doctors agree with them.

But Dr. Robert Atkins and the other "protein power" diet gurus say that *all* simple carbohydrates—whether sugar, fruit, white bread, or white rice—play havoc with your insulin production, causing you to gain weight and still feel hungry all the time. We don't need to go that far to agree that it makes sense to keep your sugar intake under control.

Fortunately, that is completely achievable with chocolate. How, you ask? What about those 25 grams of sugar? Well, for starters, 25 grams isn't all that much. Compare the sugar content of one serving of a number of common sweet products:

Milky Way Bar	35 g
100% Juice Cranberry-Grape Juice	34 g
Stonyfield Vanilla Yogurt	29 g
Ben & Jerry's Chocolate Chip Cookie Dough Ice Cream	28 g
Coca-Cola	27 g
Snapple Iced Tea	25 g
Tropicana Orange Juice	22 g

Newman's Organic Milk Chocolate Bar	20 g
Hershey's Milk Chocolate Bar	19 g
Hershey's Special Dark Bar	18 g
Entenmann's Coffee Cake	13 g
Oreos	13 g
Scharffen Berger Bittersweet Bar	10 g
Chocolove Strong Dark Chocolate Bar	9 g

We can learn a few important things from this table. One is that sugary drinks are the real problem in the American diet. Think about it: you beat yourself up over popping a few Oreos, but down that iced tea without a second thought. And note that the numbers above are for an *8-ounce serving* of drinks; the full 16-ounce bottles we tend to drink have double the sugar amount listed here.

Another conclusion we can make is that chocolate foods generally do not contribute a significant amount of calories to our diet. Estimates show chocolate to be responsible for no more than 1 percent of our calorie intake. And with the higher-quality dark chocolates, the sugar content becomes truly insignificant. The "dark chocolate" bar the USDA uses in its chart is higher in sugar and lower in cocoa content than the "good stuff." Considering that the USDA Daily Values recommend at least 300 grams of carbohydrates per day, a good dark-chocolate bar containing 9 or 10 grams isn't going to make a difference in your weight.

Cocoa Content

Looking at the ingredients list of any chocolate product can be enlightening. When you look at milk chocolate, here's what you'll probably find: sugar, milk, cocoa butter, cocoa (or chocolate), lecithin, vanilla. Yes, actual cocoa is the *fourth* ingredient. You're getting a lot more sugar and milk than you are cocoa, which explains why the health benefits of milk chocolate are so muted.

Now take a look at the ingredients of some quality dark chocolate. You will see: cocoa, sugar, cocoa butter, lecithin, vanilla. By law, dark chocolate can have only these five ingredients in it and still call itself "dark chocolate." (Of course, it can contain other flavors and ingredients and call itself "chocolate with almonds" and so on.) Here's the lowdown on each of the five ingredients:

Cocoa: Sometimes listed as cocoa liquor, this is the stuff you want, the good stuff, the real thing.

Sugar: Come on, you know what sugar is.

Cocoa Butter: This is the pure fat that occurs naturally in cacao beans. To turn cacao beans into solid or liquid chocolate, the cocoa (which has natural cocoa butter in it) is mixed with additional cocoa butter. This gives it that velvety texture and perfect melting point. (As mentioned earlier, cocoa butter seems almost as if it was designed to be popped into the human mouth. Solid at normal temperatures, it starts to soften at 75 degrees and melts at 97 degrees, which is why good chocolate turns to luscious nothingness as it sits on the tongue.)

Lecithin: This sounds like a scary preservative but is actually a useful nutrient. An emulsifier used in many foods to create a satiny, rich feel, lecithin is a lipid used to build the membranes of every cell in your body. It is particularly needed by your brain and cardiovascular system, so don't knock it. If anything, you need more lecithin (and can buy it as a nutritional supplement). Ultra-high-end chocolate makers try to get by without the lecithin, but you don't need to care much either way. Cheap chocolates may contain a lot of lecithin instead of cocoa butter, and this leads to inferior taste.

Vanilla: The Maya were adding vanilla to chocolate two thousand years ago. It's a tried-and-true flavor combination.

Obviously, the fact that cocoa is the first ingredient in serious dark chocolate and the fourth in milk chocolate means that there is a lot less cocoa in milk chocolate. Cocoa content is also regulated by the FDA. The following table shows the required cocoa content of different chocolate classifications:

Milk Chocolate	10%
Sweet Chocolate	15%
Semisweet Chocolate	15%
Bittersweet Chocolate	35%

Many "dark chocolate" products are actually bittersweet, meaning they can have three or four times the cocoa content of milk chocolate. But this is only the tip of the iceberg, because one of the encouraging recent trends in Americans' eating patterns is a tendency toward stronger and stronger chocolate. Thirty-five percent? Hah, that's nothing. Premium dark chocolate bars are routinely 55 percent cocoa or more these days. Many chocolatiers are pushing the envelope with 65 and 70 percent bars. Beyond 70 percent you run into trouble; there's so little room left for sugar and cocoa butter that you lose that melt-in-your-mouth effect. What you have, more or less, is baking chocolate: awfully good for you, but not much fun to eat straight.

Most manufacturers of these serious chocolates proudly display their cocoa content right on the labels. Think about antioxidant content as you look for cocoa percentage on a label. Considering that many of the health studies on chocolate were done with milk chocolate, or with medium-strength "dark" chocolate, you could easily be getting 2–4 times the antioxidant blast from a 70 percent bar. At that level, as much as it's food, it's also powerful medicine.

–5–

Chocolate on the Brain

*C*hocolate's reputation as a feel-good food is nothing new; after all, Montezuma wasn't pounding fifty cups a day to reduce his cholesterol levels. People have always instinctively turned to chocolate as a mood-enhancer, but in the past ten years scientists have made significant headway in understanding just why this is.

A rich brew of natural chemicals, chocolate has more than four hundred known compounds in it. Quite a few of these are psychologically active. The ones most likely responsible for chocolate's effects are caffeine, theobromine, serotonin, tryptamine, phenylethylamine, and anandamide. Let's take a look at each of these and then see if we can draw some conclusions about how they may work together to deliver that chocolate buzz.

Caffeine

We all know caffeine. The American economy practically runs on the stuff. Ninety percent of Americans drink it every day. And no wonder—caffeine really does make people more alert and productive, at least in the short run. Caffeine works by blocking the receptors in the brain that usually slow down your nerve cell activity and relax you. Influenced by caffeine, your brain's neurons begin firing more quickly. Extra dopamine is also released into your brain, giving you an emotional lift. Thinking some emergency is happening, your brain releases hormones to begin a classic "fight or flight" response: your blood pressure goes up, your heart beat increases, blood sugar level rises, your brain becomes super-alert, and blood flow is redirected from digestion and surface areas to muscles and brain instead.

All this is great if you're running from a saber-toothed tiger, or leading a board meeting. It's not so good if you want to sleep: half the caffeine you consume is still in your body six hours later. Then there is the problem of the post-caffeine crash. As the caffeine trickles out of your brain, those previously blocked receptors finally get through to you with all their fatigue messages. Neural activity plummets, muscles feel weary, heart rate drops, and on top of that you may feel depressed from the drop in dopamine. This is why, while low doses of caffeine can be great as a temporary tonic, high regular doses can cause addiction.

Fortunately, where caffeine is concerned, chocolate is not

a major player. The following table lists caffeine amounts in common products:

Coffee (12 oz)	200
Black Tea (12 oz)	140
Green Tea (12 oz)	40
Coca-Cola, Pepsi (12 oz)	50
Vivarin, Dexatrim (1 tablet)	200
No-Doz (1 tablet)	100
Anacin (1 tablet)	32
Dark Chocolate Bar (1.5 oz)	27
Milk Chocolate Bar (1.5 oz)	11

As you can see from this table, unless you are highly sensitive to caffeine and eat your brownie just before bed, the caffeine in chocolate isn't likely to throw you for a loop. After all, the average American guzzles 300 mg per day of the drug—and many people drink more than 1,000 mg.

Theobromine

Like caffeine, theobromine is a stimulant. Unlike caffeine, theobromine isn't found in a wide range of foods. Tea has a trace (about 4 mg per cup), but cocoa is the primary source of theobromine in the American diet. (The chemical was even named for the cacao plant, *Theobroma cacao*.) A bar of dark chocolate has 214 mg of theobromine, while milk chocolate has about a third of that. This makes it sound like chocolate must be an intense stimulant, but theobromine is a far milder stimulant than caffeine, packing only one-tenth the wallop. So those 214 mg of theobromine have the stimulating equivalent of 21 mg of caffeine. Adding this to the 27 mg of actual caffeine in dark chocolate, we can estimate that a 1.5-oz bar of dark chocolate has about the same stimulating effect as a can of cola.

Theobromine works slightly differently from caffeine. Most notably, it relaxes smooth muscle tissue. These milder effects may explain why people don't experience the same surge-and-crash patterns from chocolate that they get from coffee and strong tea.

Serotonin and Tryptophan

Serotonin is a neurotransmitter that regulates mood in the brain: high levels leave you calm, satisfied, and sleepy; low levels mean depression, insomnia, and poor concentration. The wildly popular antidepressant Prozac works because of its effect on serotonin levels. Prozac and the other SSRIs (selective serotonin reuptake inhibitors) inhibit the brain's ability to break down serotonin, resulting in more being present in the brain at any one time.

But drugs aren't the only way to boost serotonin levels. The body manufactures its serotonin from tryptophan, an essential amino acid found in many foods, including chocolate. Since chocolate contains some serotonin as well, you'd think that this tryptophan-serotonin one-two punch would make chocolate a first-rate sedative. But the tryptophan and serotonin levels in chocolate are pretty low. Other foods such as turkey, beans, and nuts have much more. And any sleepy effect from the tryptophan and serotonin that is present is probably offset by the mild stimulating effect of the caffeine and theobromine. There are also questions as to how well tryptophan from food makes it to the brain.

So why even mention tryptophan and serotonin? So that you won't be confused by articles that mention chocolate having these substances. Following common practices will serve you well here. If you want to sleep soundly, have a big turkey sandwich for dinner. If you want to feel happy, alert, and mellow, reach for the Godiva.

Phenylethylamine

Now things get interesting. Chocolate contains more phenylethylamine (PEA) than it does caffeine, and PEA is a powerful amphetamine cousin. Like speed and heroin, PEA triggers the release of natural opiates in the brain, which brings on feelings of ecstasy. (Eating sweet, fatty foods also releases natural opiates.) PEA is actually generated within the brain—in fact, people falling in love have a noted increase of PEA in their brains, causing it to be nicknamed the "love drug." There are sound reasons to suspect that this love drug is at least partially responsible for the good feelings derived from eating chocolate. Perhaps this even explains chocolate's popularity at

Valentine's Day—among both those in love and those who wish they were.

During orgasm, the brain is flooded with PEA. Does this explain the "better-than-sex" reputation chocolate has in some quarters? Well, before you get too excited, think about this: although PEA levels are significant in chocolate, they are far higher in salami and cheddar cheese, both of which have about ten times the PEA concentration of chocolate. Now, while many of us enjoy a good salami now and then, few have been known to sink into parox-ysms of orgasm at its consumption. Even salami cravings seem to be on the rare side. I can assure you that a Google search for "salami orgasms" brings up zero useful hits.

How could this be? Clearly, the answer is that no one chemical is responsible for chocolate's unique effect. The PEA needs help. And it gets it in anandamide.

Anandamide

Nobody knew anandamide existed until a few years ago. That was when Daniel Piomelli, a researcher at the Neurosciences Institute in San Diego, set out to discover how marijuana affects the brain. He found that the human brain produces a pleasure chemical (which he named "anandamide," after the Sanskrit word for bliss), com-pletely separate from the natural opiate system we were already familiar with, that is almost identical to the THC in marijuana. The brain has receptors for anandamide built right into it—when a molecule of anandamide "clicks" into the receptor, you get a hit of pleasure—and THC happens to fit perfectly into these receptors.

Acting on a hunch, Piomelli assumed that some potent chemical must be behind chocolate cravings, and decided to investigate. Lo and behold, he found anandamide in chocolate, making chocolate and marijuana the only known sources of these molecules.

As nervous candy companies were quick to point out, chocolate contains far lower levels of this chemical than marijuana does. You would have to eat twenty-five pounds of chocolate to get the high you get from smoking a joint. But that isn't the end of the story.

Piomelli also found two close relatives of anandamide in chocolate. Brace yourself for the names, because nobody has come up with catchy monikers for them yet: N-oleoylethanolamine and N-linoleoylethanolamine. Don't worry, you don't have to pronounce them, you just have to know what they do, which is to keep anandamide floating around the brain longer.

You see, usually anandamide has a very short lifespan in the brain. Primitive man would not have survived long if he was perpetually stoned, so your enzymes break that anandamide down as fast as it is made. But the two anandamide cousins mentioned above prevent the enzymes from doing their thing. And these cousins are found in chocolate in considerably higher levels than anandamide. This is a beautiful thing, because by prolonging the brain's natural "high," instead of flooding it with external chemicals, it's possible that chocolate delivers a much mellower and longer-lasting sense of well-being than does marijuana or other drugs. (Of course, it also means that chocolate might preserve a marijuana high, too—so that popular collegiate concoction, the marijuana brownie, might not be as random as it seems.) For this reason, scientists are now studying this effect closely, hoping that chocolate may lead them to a whole new family of effective, unintrusive antidepressants.

The Perfect Storm

Where does all this leave us? We have many promising leads, but no firm answers. Chocolate has stimulants in it, but not as much as coffee or tea. Chocolate has "love drugs" in it, but not nearly so much as cheese or salami. Chocolate has a THC-like chemical, but in minuscule quantities, though they may stick around the brain longer. And, of course, chocolate has fat and sugar in it. Then there are the hundreds of other chemicals in chocolate that may have as-yet unknown effects.

What all this adds up to is the likelihood that, while no one substance in chocolate can take the credit for its powers, the combination of mood-lifters works synergistically to create a "perfect storm" of happiness in the brain. This entire storm is what people look for when they crave chocolate, rather than any one piece of it, as we shall see.

Cravings

While the image of a depressed woman sitting at home downing mountains of chocolates is a cliché, the connection between chocolate and women's moods seems to have some basis in fact. The numbers show that chocolate is far and away the most craved food in the United States, mostly by women, and that these women have stronger cravings when they are depressed or premenstrual.

In a survey of cravings in the United States (yes, there are people paid to do such things), half of all cravings involved chocolate. And of those chocolate cravers, 75 percent said that chocolate and chocolate alone could satisfy their cravings. Overall, 40 percent of women in the United States crave chocolate, but only 15 percent of men. (Men's most-craved food? Pizza.) Most men report feeling happy after giving in to their cravings, while most women report feeling guilty.

In addition to women's chocolate cravings increasing prior to menstruation, postmenopausal women taking progesterone preparations also report developing chocolate cravings, sometimes for the first time. Some theorize that magnesium deficiencies are at the root of the PMS cravings, but lentils have more magnesium than chocolate and few premenstrual women scream for lentils.

Two recent studies have shed new light on the topic of chocolate cravings. In one, researchers surveyed college students in Spain and the United States. Sixty percent of both the Spanish and American men craved salty food or meat, while 60 percent of the women, whether Spanish or American, craved sweets. However, when asked to specify which sweets they craved, 50 percent of the American women said chocolate, while only 25 percent of the Spanish women did. If cravings for chocolate were purely a matter of biology, these numbers should be the same. Clearly, cultural factors play some part. American women are taught to satisfy their cravings with chocolate.

The second study focused on self-confessed chocoholics. When they experienced chocolate cravings, the chocoholics were given either milk chocolate, white chocolate (which contains no cocoa, only cocoa butter), a capsule filled with cocoa powder, both white chocolate and the cocoa-powder capsule, a placebo capsule, or nothing at all. The subjects were then asked whether their cravings had been satisfied. The results? Surprise! Only the milk chocolate effectively satisfied cravings. The white chocolate had some effect. The cocoa powder capsules had none. This means chocolate cravings are about taste and texture (and expectations) more than they are about PEAs, anandamide, or magnesium.

None of this defies common sense. Of course the flavor of chocolate is primary to its enjoyment. Certainly the bioactive compounds give it extra zing. Chocolate is an amazing food, but—it's important to point out—not an addictive one. Chocolate cravings are real; chocolate addiction isn't. An addiction, such as to caffeine or nicotine, is accompanied by bad physiological symptoms when the person tries to withdraw from the addiction. Headaches, shakes, nausea, depression. None of this happens if you give up chocolate. Your body doesn't get "hooked" on it. True, psychosomatic addictions can be quite strong, but people who claim they are addicted to chocolate are wrong. They could break the habit without suffering. They just don't want to. And after all, when something is as beneficial for them as chocolate, why should they?

– 6 –

Melting the Myths

$\mathscr{C}$hocolate has been a scapegoat for a long time. Though most of its history is as a health food, periodically chocolate is seized on as a source of society's ills, whether for "inciting the venereal passions" or causing apathy, indolence, or even revolutionary foment! Of course, all the same accusations have been leveled at coffee and tea, too. Rare is the exotic food that hasn't been pegged as an aphrodisiac at some point, usually with as little evidence as there is in the case of chocolate.

Following America's long Puritan tradition of believing that anything that feels really good must somehow be bad for you, we have ascribed a variety of ills to chocolate consumption. From acne and allergies to migraines and cavities, we have always found reasons to convince ourselves that we shouldn't indulge in chocolate. Most of these beliefs are built on surprisingly flimsy evidence. Let's go through the facts and put your worries to rest, one by one.

Acne

This is a biggie. Thousands of teenagers every year are *still* told to lay off the Snickers if they want those blackheads to disappear. Yet study after study has found no link between acne and food of any kind. The American Academy of Dermatologists unequivocally states that acne is not caused by diet, poor hygiene, or stress. Acne is triggered by surging testosterone levels during puberty. (Yes, girls have testosterone, too, just less of it than boys.) The surging hormones cause the oil glands in the skin to enlarge, pump out more oil, and become infected, and pizza-face is the unfortunate result. No matter how much you avoid chocolate, fat, sugar, carbohydrates, or anything else, you aren't going to be influencing this process. The best way to deal with normal acne is simply to wash your face a couple of times a day with mild soap and water.

It is interesting how long ago the myth of chocolate's connection to acne was dispelled, yet how prevalent it still is. As far back as the 1960s, researchers had shoveled piles of chocolate into willing teens and failed to trigger any acne outbreaks. Other studies throughout the 1970s and 1980s also failed to establish any role of chocolate in acne production. Today, no serious dieticians or dermatologists pay any attention to chocolate in their battle against acne. But myths die hard, and it may be decades before this particular one finally peters out.

Allergies

A lot of people seem to believe they're allergic to everything. How many people do you know who suddenly discovered they are allergic to dairy? Or wheat? Or soy? Most of these people do not have true *allergies.* What they likely have is food *intolerance,* a different and milder condition. Experts believe that only about 2 percent of adults have a true food allergy, which results when the body's immune system mistakes a protein from a food for an invading germ. When this happens, histamines are produced to fight the "invaders," and these histamines are responsible for the itchy throat, runny nose, upset stomach, and watery eyes of classic allergy symptoms. At extreme levels, the body's attack on the "invaders" can be so over-the-top that the throat closes.

Food intolerance is milder, and more common. There is no immune response, but the individual may have trouble digesting a type of food due to various reasons, such as low levels of a particular enzyme.

While most so-called wheat and dairy allergies are actually food intolerances, there are a few foods that tend to produce deadly serious allergies, peanuts and shellfish among them. Chocolate, however, is not one of these foods.

People who claim to be allergic to chocolate usually don't show any symptoms of their allergies under controlled conditions. In one study, 81 people who believed they had chocolate allergies were fed chocolate, and only 10 produced symptoms. These 10 participated in a double-blind study, and only 3 developed allergic symptoms. In another study, 20 people with "chocolate allergies" were fed capsules containing either cocoa powder (equivalent to that in an average candy bar) or a placebo. Only one seemed to have a true chocolate allergy.

ADHD

Although no one claims that chocolate is directly related to Attention-Deficit Hyperactivity Disorder (ADHD), chocolate does have sugar in it, and children particularly like chocolate, so the guilt-by-association between chocolate and "hyperactivity" is an old one. Almost all studies on ADHD, however, show no link to sugar consumption. Of twelve double-blind studies conducted between 1984 and 1994, only one showed any link between ADHD and sugar. Ten showed no link, and one showed a reduced rate of ADHD with increased sugar consumption. New information is coming to light that may point to a link between exposure to television and computer screens as an infant and ADHD. If you are worried about your child's behavior, look to his TV, not his hot chocolate.

Cavities

Sugar causes cavities, right? Are you hesitating? Has this debunking of chocolate myths got you unsure of yourself, even of something so elemental as the fact that sugar causes cavities? Well, in this case, you're right. Sugar does cause cavities. But there's more to the story than that.

Cavities are caused by bacteria in our mouths. These bacteria feed on simple carbohydrates and transform them into acid. The bacteria also combine with other substances in our food to form plaque, that sticky stuff we brush off every morning. When the bacteria and plaque stick to our teeth and produce acid, the acid weakens the enamel on our teeth, eventually "drilling" holes into the teeth that then let even more bacteria and acid in toward the nerve. Ouch.

Bacteria can use any simple carbohydrate to pull this off. That means sugar works well, but so does flour, rice, potatoes, and pasta. This is why primitive hunter-gatherer tribes, who have no agriculture and eat almost no carbohydrates, don't even have words for cavities, much less for toothbrush.

What dentists are starting to realize is that it is not the sweetness of a carbohydrate that makes it a cavity-causer, but how long it takes that food to "clear the mouth." The reality is surprising. Foods that get stuck in crevices of the mouth—such as crackers, chips, cookies, and dried fruit—are more likely to cause cavities than foods such as chocolate or soda.

Chocolate may even help prevent cavities from forming. Really. The tannins in chocolate (like those in tea and red wine) prevent bacteria from being able to form their plaque "glue" they use to stick to teeth. Research bears this out. A study of 3,000 children found no connection between chocolate consumption and cavities, and a Swedish study found that chocolate-eaters had the same rate of cavities as those who consumed no sweets at all.

Heart Palpitations

Theobroma cacao is going to have to plead guilty on this one. Many people find that they suffer heart palpitations—racing or fluttery heartbeats—after consuming caffeine in any form. While usually harmless, these palpitations can be scary and unpleasant. While chocolate has less caffeine in it than soda, tea, or coffee (see the table on page 63), and is thus less likely to cause palpitations, people who are extremely sensitive to caffeine should probably avoid chocolate as well. It's possible that the theobromine and phenylethylamine in chocolate could also contribute to heart palpitations.

Migraines

The long-standing belief that chocolate triggers migraines seems to be another case of guilt-by-association. The scenario goes like this: you've had a long, stressful day. You go home, eat some chocolate, and *wham*—a killer headache strikes. The chocolate gets blamed, but evidence shows that the headache was coming all along and the chocolate was just in the wrong place at the wrong time. Another common scenario is for women to indulge in chocolate when they are premenstrual, and to have a migraine come on at the same time. They blame the chocolate, but it turns out that women's craving for chocolate and incidence of migraine both go up when they have their periods; the two are not directly connected.

Why focus on women? Because, for reasons not completely understood, women are three times as likely to suffer from migraines and tension headaches as men, and they are more likely to crave chocolate (and other sweets) by a similar ratio.

Researchers at the University of Pittsburgh Medical Center's Pain Evaluation and Treatment Institute studied 63 women prone to migraines or tension headaches. They eliminated all suspected headache-triggers from the women's diets, then added chocolate back in to the diets of half the women, and carob, disguised as chocolate, into the diets of the other half. Chocolate was no more likely to trigger headaches than carob. Ten of these women strongly believed that chocolate triggered their migraines and were given an additional trial, yet again, chocolate consumption did not cause headaches.

A separate study of 25 migraine sufferers found the same result: women given chocolate and a carob placebo two weeks apart had no differences in their incidence of migraine.

Interestingly, some migraine research has found that women's cravings for sweets goes up prior to the onset of a migraine, so the assumed cause-effect relationship between chocolate and headaches could actually go the other way: migraines "trigger" chocolate consumption.

Obesity

"I can't eat chocolate because it will make me fat and unhealthy."

Look, if you eat three pints of chocolate ice cream per day, you're gonna get fat. For that matter, if you eat a loaf of Wonder Bread every day you're likely to get fat. Eating one serving of good-quality chocolate per day will have no impact on your weight, will improve your cholesterol, and will make you considerably less likely to get heart disease or stroke. Dieticians estimate that only 1 percent of the average American's caloric intake comes from chocolate.

Compare the 170 calories in a Scharffen Berger Bittersweet Chocolate Bar with the 750 calories in a Whopper with Cheese, the 540 calories in a large McDonald's fries, or the 570 calories in a vanilla shake. A single meal at a fast-food restaurant can easily hit the 2,000-calorie limit for an entire day's supply of food! Make your choices. Cut out the fast food, hit the Scharffen Berger, and you will be healthy, wealthy—and slim.

–7–

Chocolate Growing Today: Child Labor and Environmental Issues

*T*his is a book about health. Your personal health. But it's about much more than that. One of the most important worldwide trends is the realization that our health and well-being do not exist in a vacuum. They depend on a network of support stretching from the food we eat and the air we breathe to the stability of the nation we live in and the partners with which we trade. Eventually, this network reaches around the world and includes all the communities—human and otherwise—on this planet. Understanding this leads to the growing realization that paying the absolute cheapest price possible for a product usually results in unintended consequences that eventually come home to roost with us.

Nowhere is this more true than with the cacao industry. It seems wonderful to be able to walk into a supermarket and buy a chocolate bar for a dollar, but considering the human suffering and ecological destruction needed to make that bar cost so little, that buck comes at the future's expense.

Labor Practices

We've already seen that the original cacao industry in South America was boosted to new levels in the eighteenth century by the importation of millions of slaves from Africa. Eventually, when this practice became socially unacceptable, cacao producers got creative. They couldn't bring the labor to the trees, so they brought the trees to the labor. Vast groves of the inferior, but high-yielding, *forastero* cacao were planted throughout Africa's equatorial belt, where growing conditions were similar to those of the American tropics. The workers weren't officially slaves, but they weren't far from it, either. Wages in Africa were so low, and workers were provided with so little, that cacao could be produced cheaper and cheaper. As a result, world wholesale prices fell, and chocolate changed from an expensive luxury to an everyday staple.

Today, the situation has only become worse. African laborers are paid extraordinarily little, even by third-world standards. A Brazilian cacao laborer makes about $850 per year, which is bad enough until you compare him with his counterpart in Ivory Coast, who makes only $165. Worse, in the past few years there have been reports of abusive child labor practices in Ivory Coast, the source of 43 percent of the world's cacao. According to the reports, preteen children from Mali, a neighboring country even poorer than Ivory Coast, are forced to work twelve-hour days with no breaks on some plantations in Ivory Coast. The reports allege that some of the children are imprisoned, beaten if they don't work hard enough or try to escape, and fed a subsistence diet.

It is unclear how widespread such abuse is. A U.S. government-funded study of the situation in 2002 found very few examples of outright abuse. At the same time, the study did highlight economic issues within cacao farming that would contribute to such practices. But plantation owners are not solely to blame for this problem. We share a role in it, too. Market forces are driving the wholesale price of cacao ever lower. A truly open, global market means that producers are always competing with whoever will offer the lowest price, and if cacao producers are going to stay in business while getting less money for their product, they need to cut their own costs, and labor is the easiest place to do this.

The closer you look at the situation, the more you realize there is no easy answer. Where do you draw the line between true slavery and indentured poverty? For these cacao laborers, a poor-paying job is still better than none. And preteens working in agriculture alongside their parents has been part of African culture for centuries, if not longer. Of the one million cacao farms in West Africa, the vast majority are tiny (less than five acres) family affairs. The child labor abuses reported were confined to the few large plantations, but boycotting cacao from Ivory Coast would affect the family farms even more severely than the plantations.

To its credit, the cacao industry knows it has a potential public-relations nightmare on its hands and has established a commission to help resolve this issue as quickly as possible. But it can only do so much as long as cacao prices remain drastically low.

How far have cacao prices fallen? The drop is dizzying. Cacao today sells for *less than half* of what it sold for *thirty years ago*. For some time, the wholesale price has hovered around the current 72 cents per pound. A buyer for Ivory Coast's Society of Commercial Agricultural Producers says, "We cannot blame the farmers for exploiting these workers. The farmer has no influence on the global system. The system dictates the price."

A strong argument can be made that it is in the interest of the United States, and all of us, to help change this system. Practices that ruin the economy and social structure of poor countries can, as we've seen in the Middle East, allow unhealthy influences to develop that eventually become problems for the West, especially the United States. Paying enough to third-world farmers to allow them to lead healthy lives pays us back tenfold in our own safety and quality of life.

If you follow the recommendations I've made in this

book, you aren't eating Ivory Coast cacao anyway. Because Ivory Coast cacao is the high-yield, poorer-quality stuff, it isn't used by gourmet chocolate makers, whose high-cacao-content bars couldn't mask the flavor of inferior beans. These chocolate makers pay a premium for good-tasting beans, beans that are generally grown with better worker conditions.

Want to go a step further in support of human rights? A program called Fair Trade, which has been very successful among coffee growers, has now been extended to cacao producers, too. Fair Trade certifies producers who meet minimum social standards for their operations. In return for following these standards, Fair Trade producers receive a premium price on their beans.

Here is Fair Trade's official description of their certification standards: "There are two sets of generic producer standards, one for small farmers and one for workers on plantations and in factories. The first set applies to smallholders organized in cooperatives or other organizations with a democratic, participative structure. The second set applies to organized workers, whose employers pay decent wages, guarantee the right to join trade unions and provide good housing where relevant. On plantations and in factories, minimum health and safety as well as environmental standards must be complied with, and no child or forced labor can occur."

Look for the Fair Trade logo on chocolate products, or visit www.globalexchange.org.

Environmental Issues

Chocolate has the potential to be either an environmental calamity or a savior of the rainforest. Again, it depends on us. The calamity threat looms in Africa, where vast tracts of rainforest have been wiped out to make space for immense cacao plantations. The irony is that cacao evolved as an understory tree. It is happiest growing to heights of twenty feet in dappled shade, far below the towering tropical hardwoods. But by growing it as a monocrop in full sunlight, with acre after acre of nothing but cacao trees, producers have been able to increase yield by growing the trees much closer together than is natural, to the point where some trees are touching. Yes, this increases yield per acre, but it introduces a portfolio of problems as well.

Most important, in terms of impact, is the problem of pests and diseases. Growing naturally in the jungle, cacao trees were scattered far and wide, and even if a disease infected one tree, the chances of it spreading to another tree were slim. Not so with monocultures, where a disease, such as the dreaded witches' broom, can spread like wildfire through a grove. Says Martin Aitken, a researcher for M&M Mars in Bahia, Brazil, "Monoculture can be a very successful way of growing crops, but when it goes wrong, it goes very wrong." In recent years, cacao industries in entire countries have been destroyed by disease. Brazil's yield plunged from 400,000 tons in the 1980s to 100,000 tons today. Indonesia, Nigeria, and Malaysia have also suffered sharp declines.

To combat the heightened risk from disease and pests, monocrop plantations must use excessive amounts of pesticides, herbicides, and fungicides. This, of course, drives up costs—costs that can't be compensated by higher prices. Cacao trees also need constant water, so full-sunlight plantations must spend much more money to irrigate their trees than do understory farmers.

Overall, despite the fact that a healthy, diverse, organic cacao grove yields only about half as much fruit as a healthy monocrop of the same acreage, it can produce net profits that are 80 percent higher, due to all the money saved on fertilizers, pesticides, and irrigation, and to the higher prices paid for organic cacao.

Another, rarely cited reason for the greater success of shade-grown cacao has to do with midges. These tiny flies, which live and breed in the rich, moist leaf litter that carpets rainforest floors, are the sole pollinators of cacao flowers. When producers first created cacao groves in the open sun and saw their fertilization rates plummet, they assumed this was because the trees didn't like the full sun. But it turns out cacao trees can do fine in full sun—they just can't fertilize each other without the midges, who were left behind on the forest floor. No midges equals no fruit. This is a classic example of the unforeseen consequences that occur when people alter the incredibly complex web of interactions that mark life in the rainforest.

Even though cacao has been the impetus for massive deforestation thus far, it can still be the key to undoing much of the damage that has been done. The reason lies in its ecological niche. We know that cacao thrives best in the moist understory. And, to be painfully obvious, an understory requires an overstory. Ceiba, mahogany, and other tropical hardwoods make ideal habitat for cacao groves. Rather than seeing existing rainforest as an obstacle to agricultural production, farmers can see it as ideal habitat for cacao, and for the jobs created by cacao. True, a full-scale cacao grove will not have the same species diversity as pristine rainforest, but it is vastly better than the treeless fields that almost always replace rainforest in the tropics. By returning cacao to its rainforest home, we can turn the tide on rainforest destruction and provide a way for farmers to make their livelihoods from the living forest, removing the pressure on them to clear it for cattle or other industry.

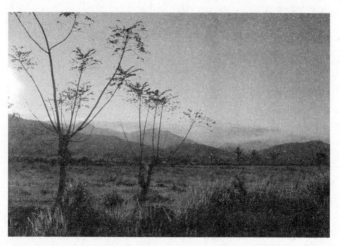

Cacao trees growing without shade in Africa.

In addition to providing an economic incentive for preserving existing rainforest, cacao could be part of a plan to regenerate rainforest where it has been cleared. Allowing overstory trees to develop in current cacao groves would take some time, and would never be a replacement for uncut, old-growth rainforest, but over decades it could lead to an economically and socially sustainable reforestation program.

For this to happen, cacao growers must switch to organic growing practices; a forest doused with fertilizer and fungicides won't ever harbor a healthy range of life forms. Since organic cacao also provides better economic conditions for its farmers, it makes sense from every angle.

We have a long way to go, however. Currently less than 1 percent of cacao is grown organically. The easy solution is market-driven: if you demand it, they will grow it. And by supporting organic chocolate companies (some of whom are listed in the Resources section) you'll also be avoiding the slave labor issues of Ivory Coast cacao; none of those producers grow organically.

I haven't even touched on the other benefit of organic cacao, the main reason most people who buy organic choose to do so: their own health. Is organic cacao better for you? Is any organic food better for you? We have no hard evidence, though we can certainly suspect that putting systemic poisons into your body is not a good idea. You bought this book, so clearly you are concerned with what goes into your body. Even if you're not concerned about rainforest health and third-world farmers' rights, you might want to play it safe and go organic.

– 8 –

Recipes

The following recipes give you all the tools you need to have chocolate for breakfast, lunch, and dinner, should you desire. Oh, and dessert too, of course. Don't get too freaked out by the number of savory chocolate recipes here. There are many places out there to find good, intense chocolate dessert recipes; there aren't many for all the other courses, so I've tried to remedy that. Don't worry, you mousse and cake lovers: you're well taken care of, too.

As I've harped on throughout this book, the key to getting the most health benefits from your chocolate is to maximize your cocoa content and minimize less healthy ingredients, particularly sugar. In keeping with that plan, I've kept the amount of sugar in these recipes quite low. If you can't take it, simply add a few more tablespoons of sugar the next time you make it.

Another way to adjust the sweetness of these recipes is to change the chocolate you use. I've called for chocolate with a 70 percent cocoa content in almost all of these, but if that turns out to be too bitter for you, you can change to 60 or 55 percent cocoa. Alternatively, you can use pure, unsweetened baking chocolate for a real blast of bitterness. If you have nothing but unsweetened chocolate on hand and you want to follow these recipes, add 3 tablespoons of sugar per ounce of chocolate.

Chocolate Sauce

This ultra-simple sauce has a million uses. Here's one: use it as a dip for tortilla chips. You'll be amazed. It also keeps forever in the fridge, so make plenty and use it daily. Depending on the primary ways you use it, you can choose to make it with unsweetened chocolate or cocoa powder and just add 3 tablespoons of extra sugar per ounce of sauce in recipes. It can be handy for this recipe to use the packages of little chocolate disks now sold by various companies, including Dagoba.

8 oz   70% chocolate, chopped
5 T   canola oil
2 T   vanilla extract

1. Heat the oil over low heat in a small saucepan.
2. Add the chocolate and mix, stirring constantly, until melted and silky. Mix in the vanilla.
3. Ladle over your entire life.

Chocolate Tandoori

Tandoori is a traditional cooking style of India in which meats are marinated in a yogurt-spice mixture and then baked over high heat in a clay oven (a tandoor). Indian and Mexican cuisine share many elements, and many of the classic spices of Asia have been used with chocolate since the seventeenth century, so this combination really doesn't range that far afield. The chocolate and spices impart the meat with an intense earthiness, and the yogurt lends a creaminess to the chocolate. For a truly Maya meal, make this with guinea pig. If you don't have a guinea pig handy, chicken or tofu will suffice.

For marinade:

¼	c	fresh lemon juice
½	c	plain yogurt
3	T	cocoa powder
2	t	cayenne
1	T	peeled and minced fresh ginger
1	t	ground coriander
¼	t	cloves
¼	t	nutmeg
¼	t	black pepper
1	t	salt
4		boneless, skinless chicken breasts, or firm tofu slices
2	T	vegetable oil

1. Blend all marinade ingredients to a paste in a food processor or mix by hand.
2. Cut several diagonal slits in each piece of chicken or tofu, about ¼-inch deep. Cover with the marinade and marinate at least 2 hours in the refrigerator.
3. Preheat broiler.
4. Brush broiling rack with oil. Arrange chicken or tofu on rack. Brush with oil. Broil about 3 inches from the heat for approximately 7 minutes. Turn over and brush with remaining oil. Cook an additional 6 minutes, until cooked through but not dried out.

Serves 4

Chocolate Corn Bread

Ah, that sainted corn-chocolate combination! If you already have a favorite corn bread recipe, just sprinkle a couple of tablespoons of cocoa powder into the batter to get the desired effect. If not, try this one. Use a jalapeno pepper for an added splash of Mexico.

2	c	yellow cornmeal
1	c	unbleached white flour
1	c	whole wheat flour
3	T	cocoa powder
2	T	baking powder
1	t	salt
2		eggs
2	c	buttermilk
8	T	canola oil
1		jalapeno pepper, minced (optional)

1. Preheat the oven to 400° F.
2. Stir together the cornmeal, flour, cocoa powder, baking powder, and salt in a large bowl.
3. In another bowl, mix together the eggs, buttermilk, and all but 2 tablespoons of the oil.
4. Add the remaining two tablespoons of oil to a 10-inch cast-iron skillet and set in the oven. Let this heat up enough to get quite hot, but not hot enough to smoke. The goal is to sear a good crust onto your corn bread right away.

5. While the skillet is heating, stir the wet ingredients into the dry ingredients. Add the jalapeno pepper, if desired.

6. Pull the skillet from the oven, pour the batter into it, and bake for about 25 minutes, until a toothpick inserted into the center comes out clean.

7. Remove from the oven and allow the cornbread to sit for 15 minutes before removing. Serve as a side dish, or straight up with butter or honey.

Mary's Holy Mole

My wife Mary makes this mole. It's a fair amount of work, so she has to be coaxed into it, but once she does, word spreads through our town that mole is in the works. People show up unexpectedly, and the whole event turns into a sort of Mesoamerican ceremony (minus the human sacrifices). Really, it doesn't get any better than mole. The depth of flavor, the combination of the dried peppers, chocolate, nuts, and onions, the versatility of the sauce— this is the time to break out the tequila and call in sick the next morning.

In the States we tend to think of mole as a sauce for turkey or chicken, but Mexicans make the sauce ahead of time, freeze it, and use it with a wide variety of meats and vegetables. Use your imagination; you can't possibly go wrong.

12		dried ancho chiles
½	c	raisins
8		cloves garlic, unpeeled
1		large onion, unpeeled
½	c	sesame seeds
½	c	almonds
3	oz	70% chocolate, chopped
1	t	cinnamon
1	t	oregano
		salt and pepper to taste

1. Stem and seed the chiles. Heat a cast-iron skillet over medium heat and toast chiles for about 1 minute on each side. Transfer chiles to a large bowl, add raisins, and cover with hot water. Soak for 30 minutes.
2. Toast the unpeeled garlic and onion in the skillet until blackened, about 6 minutes. Set aside to cool.
3. Toast the sesame seeds and almonds in the skillet for 30 seconds. Do not let them burn. Set aside to cool.
4. Drain the chiles and raisins, reserving the soaking liquid. Put in a blender with 1 cup of the liquid.
5. Peel the garlic and onion and add to the blender.
6. Add the sesame seeds and almonds and blend the mixture into a paste, adding more soaking liquid if necessary.
7. Pour the paste into the skillet and heat over medium heat.
8. Add the chocolate, cinnamon, and oregano. Cook, stirring, for 10 to 15 minutes, until flavors are well married.
9. Correct seasoning and serve immediately as a sauce or freeze for later use.

Makes 2 cups paste

Sicilian Chocolate Pasta

Fish and chocolate? You shudder, I know, but there is great tradition behind this one. Italian chefs pushed the envelope in the 1700s and came up with a version of this rich, luscious sauce. And a Maya bowl from the sixth century was recently found in Honduras with residues of chocolate and fish bones in it. In a way, this isn't that far from Mexican mole. Both dishes use chiles, nuts, chocolate, onions, raisins, and some sort of meat. And both will leave you in a cloud of flavor-overload bliss. Vegetarians can leave out the sardines, increase the nuts, and still achieve divine results.

½	c	almond oil
1		medium onion, chopped
1		can sardines
1		bulb fennel, chopped
½	c	almonds, chopped
½	c	pine nuts
¼	c	raisins
½	c	chocolate sauce (see p. 91)
1	lb	spaghetti or other long pasta

1. Bring a large pot of salted water to a boil.
2. While waiting for the water to boil, preheat the oven to 300° F.
3. Spread the pine nuts and chopped almonds on a baking sheet and bake in the oven until toasted and lightly

browned, about 5 minutes. Watch carefully, as they can quickly burn. Remove from oven and set aside.

4. Heat almond oil in a large skillet. Add onions and fennel and sauté until soft.

5. Add sardines, almonds, pine nuts, and raisins and cook over medium heat until flavors have mixed and deepened, about 10 minutes.

6. Reduce heat, add chocolate sauce, mix well, and cook until hot, about 5 minutes.

7. Meanwhile, add the spaghetti to the boiling water and boil until *al dente,* about 6 minutes. Drain.

8. Coarsely chop the fennel fronds.

9. Top the spaghetti with the sauce, garnish with the fennel fronds, and serve at once.

Serves 4–6

New World Nachos

Many of the typical nacho ingredients, such as corn, beans, avocados, and tomatoes, are foods that have been staples of the people of Mesoamerica for centuries. The part of nachos that is unquestionably an old-world addition is the cheese. The Maya and Aztecs didn't eat any dairy products. But switch the cheese for some equally gooey, barely sweet chocolate sauce, and you have the perfect New World Super Bowl snack. Serve it at your next Maya ball game.

	10 oz tortilla chips
1	14-oz can black beans, drained
1	avocado, chopped
	8 oz prepared salsa
½ c	frozen corn kernels
1 c	chocolate sauce (see p. 91), gently warmed

1. Preheat over to 350° F.
2. Spread tortilla chips on a baking sheet. Cover them with the beans, avocado, salsa, and corn.
3. Bake in the oven until hot, about 12 minutes.
4. Remove the nachos from the oven, top with the chocolate sauce, and serve.

Serves 4 as a first course

Chocolate Breakfast Atole

For millennia, Mesoamericans have consumed drinks called *atoles* that are related to oatmeal or porridge. Thickened with corn flour, and thinner than traditional porridge, so that they can be drunk without an extra utensil, *atoles* are drunk at many times of day. In the United States, they probably work best as a breakfast-in-a-mug, and are vastly more satisfying than the breakfast drinks many of us consume. This chocolate *atole* will fortify you for a whole morning.

2 T   masa harina (corn flour)
      pinch cinnamon
      pinch salt
2 c   skim milk
1 oz 70% chocolate, finely chopped

1. Mix the masa harina, cinnamon, salt, and 1 cup of the milk in a saucepan and cook, stirring, until the mixture becomes thick and translucent. Set aside.
2. Heat the remaining cup of milk in another saucepan and add the chocolate, stirring until the mixture is smooth.
3. Add the chocolate mixture to the masa mixture and stir well. Serve immediately in mugs.

Serves 2

Grown-up Hot Chocolate

Forget Swiss Miss; this is something to save until the kids have gone to bed. Real hot chocolate, in the Maya tradition, should be rich, thick, aromatic, and spicy. It blows away any after-dinner liqueur you can think of, believe me. Those cultures that have gotten serious about their chocolate drinking—the Maya, Aztecs, Spanish—all agree that the drink is best frothed to produce a good, foamy head. There are a few ways to accomplish this. The Maya poured the drink back and forth between two cups. A bit time-consuming and messy, perhaps? The Spanish improved on this by using *molinillos,* wooden sticks with ridges or rings on one end. They would twirl these vigorously between their palms, creating quite a froth in no time. Mexican cooks use *molinillos* to this day. I prefer the frothers available in any good kitchen store. Shaped like miniature French-press coffee carafes, and intended for frothing milk for cappuccino, they make gorgeous chocolate froth.

2 c	whole milk
2 oz	60–70% chocolate, grated or chopped
¼ t	vanilla extract
¼ t	cinnamon
	pinch salt
¼ t	cayenne powder (optional)

1. Heat the milk in a saucepan until it is simmering.
2. Mix in the chocolate, stirring constantly until blended.

3. Add the vanilla, cinnamon, salt, and cayenne (if using). Heat for another minute.
4. Froth the heck out of the drink, using whatever method you prefer.
5. Serve in warm mugs.

Serves 2

Righteous Cookies

You can be righteous about these chocolate-chip cookies because they have half the sugar of common recipes, whole wheat flour, and a little extra chocolate. They are basically health food—egg for protein, complex carbohydrates, and plenty of antioxidants from the chocolate. I find that you can cut the amount of sugar in half in most recipes you see, and no one will ever notice.

1		stick butter, softened
½	c	sugar
1		egg
1	t	vanilla
1	c	unbleached white flour
1	c	whole wheat flour
½	t	baking soda
¼	t	salt
1 ½	c	70% chocolate, chips or chopped

1. Preheat the oven to 350° F. Grease your cookie sheets.
2. Cream the butter and sugar together in a large bowl. Mix in the egg and vanilla.
3. In another bowl, mix together the flours, baking soda, and salt.
4. Mix the dry ingredients into the wet ingredients. Stir in the chocolate.
5. Drop the dough onto the cookie sheets, one mounded tablespoon per cookie. Cook 10 to 12 minutes, until

golden brown. Remember, it's always better to under-
bake cookies than to overbake them.

6. Remove the sheets and let them cool for a couple of
   minutes. The cookies will firm up. Then, using a spatula, transfer them to cooling racks or a brown paper bag.

Makes 2 dozen cookies

Not-Messing-Around Chocolate Cake

As the title implies, this recipe is serious. It comes from Tara Hamilton, a woman known far and wide for the extraordinary meals that take place at her mountain home in Warren, Vermont. What I like about this one is the complete lack of flour (useless carbs) and the minimal sugar content. You will know you are eating chocolate when you bite into this dense, rich extravagance—so use your very best.

1 lb	70% chocolate (chopped or disks)
1 ½	sticks unsalted butter
2 T	kirsch, or other liqueur
6	eggs
½ c	sugar
1 c	whipping cream
	pinch cinnamon

1. Butter and flour a 9-inch-diameter springform pan.
2. Melt the chocolate and the butter together in a double boiler or saucepan over low heat, stirring constantly, until smooth. Remove from heat.
3. Preheat the oven to 350° F.
4. Beat the eggs, sugar, and kirsch together with a mixer for about 3 minutes.
5. Mix the chocolate sauce into the egg mixture until smooth. Pour the batter into the springform pan.
6. Bake the cake in the oven for about 50 minutes, until a

tester inserted into the center comes out clean. Remove from the oven and let cool. Run a knife around the sides to free the cake, then pop the sides of the springform pan loose.

7. Pour the cream in a bowl, add the cinnamon, and whip with an electric beater until stiff.

8. Serve the cake in small wedges topped with the cinnamon cream.

Serves 12

World's Best Brownies

What book on chocolate would be complete without a good brownie recipe? And this is a good one. What I like about it is the intense chocolate flavor, the relatively low sugar content, and the fact that it uses whole wheat flour, which is much kinder to the body. The optional rum is pretty kind, too. Another option: toss in some cayenne pepper for a kick the Aztecs would have been right at home with.

1		stick butter
5	oz	unsweetened chocolate, grated or chopped
1	c	sugar
2	t	vanilla extract
2		eggs
1	c	whole wheat flour
1	T	dark rum (optional)
1	T	cayenne (optional)

1. Preheat the oven to 350° F.
2. Grease a 9-inch square cake pan.
3. In a large saucepan, melt the butter over low heat, add the chocolate, and stir constantly until melted and smooth. Remove from the heat. Let cool a few minutes before the next step.
4. Mix in the sugar, vanilla, eggs, flour, rum (if using), and cayenne (if using). Stir well until all ingredients are thoroughly mixed.

5. Bake in the oven for about 30 minutes, until a toothpick inserted into the center comes out clean.
   Remember, underbaking is better than overbaking.
6. Let cool, then cut into squares and serve.

Makes 16 brownies

Simple Chocolate Mousse

Mousse is one of the purest presentations of chocolate. It calls for your best chocolate, because with no other flavors around to hide behind, the flavor of the chocolate (and the lightness of the texture) is what makes or breaks the dish. This is a great recipe to try with different chocolates, to begin to get a sense of their unique tastes. Make mousses well ahead of time, so they have time to chill.

¼ c	light cream or half-and-half
5	eggs, separated
8 oz	70% chocolate, chopped or grated
1 T	vanilla extract
	pinch salt
1 c	whipping cream

1. Mix the cream and egg yolks together and cook over low heat until thickened but not boiling. Remove from heat and whisk in chocolate and vanilla until smooth and silky. Set aside and let cool.
2. Beat the egg whites and salt in a separate bowl until soft peaks form.
3. Gently fold the egg whites into the chocolate mixture. Don't overmix; the goal is to keep as much air in the mix as possible.
4. Pour the mousse into individual wine or parfait glasses and chill in the fridge for 6 hours (overnight works, too).

5. Before serving, pour the cream in a bowl, and whip with an electric beater until stiff.

6. Dollop the glasses of mousse with whipped cream. If the occasion is fancy, chocolate shavings over the top are an especially nice touch.

Serves 8

Enrobed Bananas

Enrobing is the process of covering candies in a coat of chocolate. Here, bananas are blanketed in warm chocolate sauce. It's basically a banana split without the ice cream, and as such is healthy all-around, so to speak.

    ½ c   almonds, finely chopped
    2   ripe bananas
    ½ c   chocolate sauce (see p. 91)
    1 c   whipping cream
          pinch cinnamon
          fresh cherries, for garnish

1. Preheat the oven to 300° F.
2. Spread the chopped almonds on a baking sheet and bake in the oven until toasted and lightly browned, about 5 minutes. Watch carefully, as they can quickly burn. Remove from oven and set aside.
3. Split the bananas lengthwise and place two halves in each of two bowls.
4. Cover generously with the chocolate sauce.
5. Scatter the toasted almonds over the top.
6. Pour the cream in a bowl, add the cinnamon, and whip with an electric beater until stiff.
7. Top the bananas with the whipped cinnamon cream and cherries and serve.

Serves 2

Conclusion

Chocolate Is Not Sinful

Is chocolate a miracle drug that will cure all your ills and keep you in a state of bliss to the ripe old age of a hundred and ten? Of course not. Though I've been eager to trumpet the many healing powers of chocolate in this book, I hope you have seen that chocolate is best used in conjunction with many other natural foods as part of an all-around healthy diet. If I achieve one thing with this book, I hope it is to separate chocolate from the myths and taboos that have surrounded it for centuries, from the guilt that so often rides with it, and to once again let it be seen as the gift from the rainforest that it is.

Our bodies instinctively respond to foods that are good for us. Infants adore the taste of mother's milk, and few adults can turn away an ultra-ripe tomato drizzled with olive oil. True, decades of bad diets have tricked us into thinking we want super-sugary desserts and salty French fries, but when our bodies scream out cravings as intently as they do for chocolate, we had better listen to them and see what they're saying.

What they seem to be saying, and what science is confirming, is that chocolate in moderation really can help us live longer, healthier, and happier. This is a good thing, and this knowledge adds so much to the already scrumptious experience of eating chocolate that it would be a crime to not let everyone in on the news.

So spread the word. Don't let diet police with information twenty years out of date, or others whose job is to make you feel bad, stop you from having a great human experience that people have been indulging in for three thousand years. Chocolate is good. Eat it as close to its natural state as possible, with just enough sugar mixed in to make it go down easy, and remind yourself that you are doing exactly what you should be.

The World's Healthiest, Most Delicious Chocolate, Delivered to Your Door

Chocolate Companies

The following companies have been singled out because they all offer serious chocolate with high cocoa content, allowing you to get maximum antioxidant value. They are also all distributed throughout the United States. Many regional chocolate makers offer fantastic chocolates as well; seek them out.

Special mention is made here for companies offering organic chocolates for two reasons. First, organic means you are getting beans that haven't been sprayed with pesticides, from groves where the trees are tended in ways that enrich the forest, rather than deplete it. Second, almost none of the large-scale, poor-quality *forastero* plantations of Africa use organic methods, so by choosing organic chocolate you are virtually assuring yourself of getting the good stuff—*criollo* or *trinitario* beans, usually from the Caribbean, Madagascar, Belize, or Venezuela. The knock against many organic foods is that they don't taste any different than the cheaper kind, but in chocolate the difference is *real*—organic really does taste better. It's also worth seeking out chocolate with the Fair Trade logo, which means the cacao farmers were paid a livable wage for their crop.

Bonnat

www.bonnat-chocolatier.com

Chocolate gourmets the world over make the pilgrimage to the Bonnat factory in Voiron, France, to sample the delights of this chocolate maker who has been in business since 1884. Bonnat's line of 75%, single-origin chocolates are about as serious as it gets. The Chuao, Madagascar, and Puerto Cabello bars are excellent quality and amazingly unique.

Chocolove

303-786-7888

www.chocolove.com

This Boulder, Colorado company imports all their chocolate bars from Belgium, and offers them in a range from 33% to 77% cocoa. They also offer organic 61% and 73% bars made exclusively from Caribbean beans, which present superb richness without overpowering bitterness.

Michel Cluizel

This famed French chocolatier does not sell directly, but may just make the best chocolate in the world. Certainly the two "premiere cru" bars—Hacienda Concepcion and Hacienda Los Ancones—are as good as it gets. Worth seeking out from a number of websites and mail order catalogs.

Cocoa Camino

613-235-6122

www.lasiembra.com

This Swiss company produces 100% organic, Fair Trade chocolate grown by a small farmer cooperative in the Dominican Republic. It also uses Fair Trade sugarcane. Its products include a 38% milk chocolate bar, a 55% dark chocolate with almonds, a 71% bittersweet bar, and cocoa powder.

Dagoba

541-664-9030

www.dagobachocolate.com

Like Cocoa Camino, Dagoba, in Oregon, makes chocolate and cocoa powder that is organic and Fair Trade grown by the Conacado cooperative in the Dominican Republic. Bars range from 59% to 74% cocoa.

El Rey

800-357-3999

www.chocolate-elrey.com

With the exception of the Grenada Chocolate Company, El Rey is manufactured as close to the source as you can get. While companies in the United States or Europe take months to ship their beans from the plantations to the factory, El Rey is in Venezuela and uses only high-quality local beans for its chocolates, which range from a 41% milk chocolate to the intense 73.5% Apamate bar, which contains extra cocoa butter for a dark, rustic, yet intensely smooth experience. Family-owned since 1929, El Rey is a chocolate institution.

Green & Black's
401-683-3323
www.greenandblacks.com

This British company makes a variety of organic chocolate products that are well-distributed in the United States. They also work with a Maya cooperative in Belize to produce Maya Gold, a 55% cocoa bar flavored with orange, cinnamon, nutmeg, and vanilla—the first commercial cacao produced by the Maya in several hundred years.

Grenada Chocolate Company
473-442-0050
www.grenadachocolate.com

You've got to like everything about the Grenada Chocolate Company, from their colorful Caribbean packaging to their commitment to using local beans and paying local workers good wages. Most of all, you've got to like their 60% and 74% dark chocolate bars and their Sweetypods—the Caribbean's answer to Hershey's Kisses, individually wrapped to look like tiny cacao pods. Their tiny factory is right in the rainforest where the cacao is grown, and they have formed a cooperative with the farmers, giving them the most direct relationship to the groves of any chocolate maker on the planet. As if that wasn't enough, their entire factory is solar-powered, giving new meaning to the term *sustainable agriculture*. The island of Grenada produces some of the finest *trinitario* and *criollo* cacao in the world, so you can't go wrong with this exemplary small company.

Lindt

This Swiss chocolate giant—one of the largest chocolate companies in the world—makes a lot of chocolates that seem dark until you taste *real* dark chocolate, but they now make some very serious bars as well. Called "Excellence," these include a 70% bar and a super-dark 85% bar that, since it uses the antioxidant-rich *forastero* beans, may just be one of the healthiest bars on the planet. These bars are more widely distributed than many of the chocolates mentioned in this section, so look for them at your local supermarket or pharmacy.

M&M Mars

www.cocoapro.com

What are *these* guys doing in this section, you ask? Not because they make chocolates that are high in healthy cocoa and low in sugar, but because they have invented a process called CocoaPro that maximizes the amount of flavonoids in chocolate. Flavonoids are usually partially destroyed by the fermenting and roasting processes that beans go through, but they are less affected by the CocoaPro system. Look for the CocoaPro logo on labels—but remember that even Dove Dark doesn't have nearly the cocoa content of the more serious chocolates listed in this section.

Scharffen Berger

800-930-4528

www.scharffenberger.com

The only American chocolate maker founded in the past fifty years, Scharffen Berger opened in 1996 in Berkeley, California, where they make high-quality chocolates on vintage European equipment. They blend beans from Indonesia, Venezuela, Madagascar, Ghana, and the Caribbean into 62% and 70% bars, as well as a number of other products (including an all-natural chocolate perfume!).

Valrhona

310-277-0441

www.valrhona.com

The Rolls Royce of chocolate, this French firm is as high-class as it gets. There are too many products to identify here—everything you can think of, they make—but worth special mention are the Grand Cru bars coming from single chocolate estates in Venezuela, Trinidad, Madagascar, and elsewhere, usually with about a 65% cocoa content. The 70% Guanaja is particularly fine.

Mail Order

Chocosphere

877-992-4626

www.chocosphere.com

Why bother going anywhere else? This incredible
Internet site sells chocolates from Valrhona, El Rey, Michel
Cluizel, Scharffen Berger, Dagoba, the Grenada Chocolate
Company, and many other top-notch sources, and has a
state-of-the-art ordering system on its website. It will
even ship your chocolate in special insulated containers to
prevent meltage during summer months.

Echocolates

1-800-207-7058

www.echocolates.com

This guys knows his chocolate. If Echocolates doesn't
have it, it probably isn't available. Echocolates distributes
1,500 different chocolate products, supports small growers, is devoted to social and environmental responsibility,
and has a wealth of chocolate information on its sight.
Not a bad idea to make this your first stop in any chocolate hunt.

2311 Gourmet

800-626-9463

www.2311gourmet.com

Well, one reason you might want to bother going some-
where else other than Chocosphere is because this gourmet

food branch of Los Angeles's leading wine purveyor carries the complete line of Bonnat chocolates, perhaps the most famed chocolatier in Paris. For $37 you can get a set of the seven Bonnat bars, each a single-estate chocolate from a different region. For $30 you can get each of Michel Cluizel's seven bars.

Magazines

Chocolatier
212-239-0855
45 West 34th St., Suite 600
New York, NY 10001

The premiere magazine devoted to chocolate, featuring a treasure trove of recipes and information in every issue.

Informational Websites

Chocolate Information Center
www.chocolateinfo.com

Go here for more information on chocolate and health than you ever wanted to know (and even more than is in this book!). The site is supported by Mars, which should raise suspicions, but it's careful to simply summarize the many scientific articles being published on chocolate's health benefits. Extremely in-depth coverage.

World Cocoa Foundation

www.chocolateandcocoa.org

A joint venture of the American Cocoa Research Institute, the Chocolate Manufacturers Association, the National Confectioners Association, and some of the largest chocolate companies in the world, this site is a gold mine of all things chocolate. It's particularly fine on nutrition and health, history, and current industry issues. It's industry-supported, but the information on the site seems to be quite accurate.

Global Exchange

www.globalexchange.org

Provides information on Fair Trade certification for cacao and coffee, and includes lists of chocolate companies using Fair Trade cacao.

Acknowledgments

Thanks first and foremost to Invisible Cities Press publisher Michael Grimaldi, for not raising his eyebrow too high when I said, "It's good for you. Really," and for seeing the need to get the word out. And for being able to tell a Bonnat from a Cluizel with his eyes closed.

Thanks to Peter Holm for the snappy design and for being a rock at all times. Thanks to Mary Elder Jacobsen and Susannah Noel for showing me my blind spots and being sticklers for details. And thanks to Tia McCarthy for her perfect taste in all matters.

Thanks to Cathi Buni, Dan Eckstein, Deb Fleischman, Michelle Morris, Liza Walker, and Nat Winthrop for enduring some of the wonkiest sections of this book and giving me valuable feedback.

I'd also like to acknowledge Sophie and Michael Coe's book *The True History of Chocolate*. This incredible work of scholarship is far and away the definitive word on the origins of the "food of the gods," as well as its development right up through the twentieth century. All who have educated themselves on the history of chocolate owe the Coes their gratitude.

And last, thanks to Eric, for liking the dark stuff from the very beginning.

References

Arts I, Hollman P, and Kromhouf D. "Chocolate as a Source of Tea Flavonoids." *The Lancet* 354 (August 7, 1999): 488.

Brenner J. *The Emperors of Chocolate*. New York: Random House, 1999.

Bright C. "Chocolate Could Bring the Forest Back." *World Watch* (November/December 2001): 17–28.

"Chalk One Up for Chocolate." *UC Berkeley Wellness Letter* (April 1999): 8.

Chang K. "Before Kisses and Snickers, It Was the Treat of Royalty." *The New York Times* (June 10, 2003).

"Chocolate and Health." *Chocolate Manufacturer's Association*. www.candyusa.org (January 15, 2003).

"Chocolate 'Could Cure Coughs.'" *BBC News*. www.bbc.com (March 3, 2003).

"The Chocolate Paradox." *Scharffen Berger Chocolate Maker*. www.scharffenberger.com (January 22, 2003).

"Chocolate: As Hearty as Red Wine." *Science News* 150 (October 12, 1996): 235.

"The CocoaPro Process." *CocoaPro*. www.cocoapro.com (February 2, 2003).

Coe S and M. *The True History of Chocolate*. New York: Thames and Hudson, 2000.

De Las Nueces D. "Yet Another Reason to Eat Chocolate." *The New York Times* (August 10, 1999): F8.

diTomaso E, Beltramo M, and Piomelli D. "Brain Cannabinoids in Chocolate." *Nature* 382 (August 22, 1996): 677.

"Eat Sweets, Live Longer." *Science News Online,* www.sciencenews.org (January 15, 2003).

"Flavanols and Chocolate." *Chocolate Information Center*. www.chocolateinfo.com (January 17, 2003).

Kim H and Keeney P. "(-)Epicatechin Content in Fermented and Unfermented Cocoa Beans." *Journal of Food Science* 49 (1984): 1080.

Kris-Etherton P, Derr J, and Mitchell D. "The Role of Fatty Acid Saturation on Plasma Lipids, Lipoproteins and Apoliproteins. Effects of Whole Food Diets High in Cocoa Butter, Olive Oil, Soybean Oil, Dairy Butter and Milk Chocolate on the Plasma Lipids of Young Men." *Metabolism* 42 (1993): 130–34.

Kris-Etherton P, et al. "A Milk Chocolate Bar/Day Substituted for a High Carbohydrate Snack Increases High-Density Lipoprotein Cholesterol in Young Men on a NCEP/AHA Step One Diet." *American Journal of Clinical Nutrition* 60 (1994): 1037S–42S.

McCord H. "Is Chocolate a Vegetable?" *Prevention* (March 1997): 51.

Ono Y. "Polyphenols Put Sparkle in Japanese Sales." *The Wall Street Journal* (March 24, 1999): B9.

Parnes R. "How Antioxidants Work." *How Stuff Works*. www.how-stuffworks.com (January 10, 2003).

"Prescription-Strength Chocolate." *Science News Online*. www.sci-encenews.org (October 12, 1996).

Presilla M. *The New Taste of Chocolate.* Berkeley, CA: Ten Speed, 2001.

Raghavan S and Chatterjee S. "Slave Labor Taints Sweetness of World's Chocolate." *Kansas City Star* (June 23, 2001).

Raloff J. "Have Danes Solved the French Paradox?" *Science News* 149 (March 30, 1996).

Raloff J. "Chocolate Hearts." *Science News* 157 (March 18, 2000).

Rein D, et al. "Cocoa Inhibits Platelet Activation and Function." *American Journal of Clinical Nutrition* 72 (2000): 30–35.

Schramm D, et al. Chocolate Procyanidins Decrease the Leukotriene/Prostacyclin Ratio in Humans and Human Aortic Endothelial Cells." *American Journal of Clinical Nutrition* 73 (2001): 36–40.

Steinberg F, Bearden M, and Keen C. "Cocoa and Chocolate Flavonoids: Implications for Cardiovascular Health." *Journal of the American Dietetic Association* 103 (2003): 215–23.

Wan Y, et al. "Effects of Cocoa Powder and Dark Chocolate on LDL Oxidative Susceptibility and Prostaglandin Concentrations in Humans." *American Journal of Clinical Nutrition* 74 (2001): 596–602.

Waterhouse A, Shirley J, and Donovan J. "Antioxidants in Chocolate." *The Lancet* 348 (September 21, 1996): 834.